Cervix Cancer

Cancer Treatment and Research

WILLIAM L MCGUIRE, *series editor*

Livingston RB (ed): Lung Cancer 1. 1981. ISBN 90-247-2394-9.
Bennett Humphrey G, Dehner LP, Grindey GB, Acton RT (eds): Pediatric Oncology 1. 1981. ISBN 90-247-2408-2.
DeCosse JJ, Sherlock P (eds): Gastrointestinal Cancer 1. 1981. ISBN 90-247-2461-9.
Bennett JM (ed): Lymphomas 1, including Hodgkin's Disease. 1981. ISBN 90-247-2479-1.
Bloomfield CD (ed): Adult Leukemias 1. 1982. ISBN 90-247-2478-3.
Paulson DF (ed): Genitourinary Cancer 1. 1982. ISBN 90-247-2480-5.
Muggia FM (ed): Cancer Chemotherapy 1. ISBN 90-247-2713-8.
Bennett Humphrey G, Grindey GB (eds): Pancreatic Tumors in Children. 1982. ISBN 90-247-2702-2.
Costanzi JJ (ed): Malignant Melanoma 1. 1983. ISBN 90-247-2706-5.
Griffiths CT, Fuller AF (eds): Gynecologic Oncology. 1983. ISBN 0-89838-555-5.
Greco AF (ed): Biology and Management of Lung Cancer. 1983. ISBN 0-89838-554-7.
Walker MD (ed): Oncology of the Nervous System. 1983. ISBN 0-89838-567-9.
Higby DJ (ed): Supportive Care in Cancer Therapy. 1983. ISBN 0-89838-569-5.
Herberman RB (ed): Basic and Clinical Tumor Immunology. 1983. ISBN 0-89838-579-2.
Baker LH (ed): Soft Tissue Sarcomas. 1983. ISBN 0-89838-584-9.
Bennett JM (ed): Controversies in the Management of Lymphomas. 1983. ISBN 0-89838-586-5.
Bennett Humphrey G, Grindey GB (eds): Adrenal and Endocrine Tumors in Children. 1983. ISBN 0-89838-590-3.
DeCosse JJ, Sherlock P (eds): Clinical Management of Gastrointestinal Cancer. 1984. ISBN 0-89838-601-2.
Catalona WJ, Ratliff TL (eds): Urologic Oncology. 1984. ISBN 0-89838-628-4.
Santen RJ, Manni A (eds): Diagnosis and Management of Endocrine-related Tumors. 1984. ISBN 0-89838-636-5.
Costanzi JJ (ed): Clinical Management of Malignant Melanoma. 1984. ISBN 0-89838-656-X.
Wolf GT (ed): Head and Neck Oncology. 1984. ISBN 0-89838-657-8.
Alberts DS, Surwit EA (eds): Ovarian Cancer. 1985. ISBN 0-89838-676-4.
Muggia FM (ed): Experimental and Clinical Progress in Cancer Chemotherapy. 1985. ISBN 0-89838-679-9.
Higby DJ (ed): The Cancer Patient and Supportive Care. 1985. ISBN 0-89838-690-X.
Bloomfield CD (ed): Chronic and Acute Leukemias in Adults. 1985. ISBN 0-89838-702-7.
Herberman RB (ed): Cancer Immunology: Innovative Approaches to Therapy. 1986. ISBN 0-89838-757-4.
Hansen HH (ed): Lung Cancer: Basic and Clinical Aspects. 1986. ISBN 0-89838-763-9.
Pinedo HM, Verweij J (eds): Clinical Management of Soft Tissue Sarcomas. 1986. ISBN 0-89838-808-2.
Higby DJ (ed): Issues in Supportive Care of Cancer Patients. 1986. ISBN 0-89838-816-3.
Surwit EA, Alberts DS (eds): Cervix Cancer. 1987. ISBN 0-89838-822-8.
Jacobs C (ed): Cancers of the Head and Neck. 1987. ISBN 0-89838-825-2.
MacDonald JS (ed): Gastrointestinal Oncology. 1987. ISBN 0-89838-829-5.
Ratliff TL, Catalona WJ (eds): Genitourinary Cancer. 1987. ISBN 0-89838-830-9.
Nathanson L (ed): Basic and Clinical Aspects of Malignant Melanoma. 1987. ISBN 0-89838-856-2.
Muggia FM (ed): Concepts, Clinical Developments, and Therapeutic Advances in Cancer Chemotherapy. 1987. ISBN 0-89838-879-5.

Cervix Cancer

edited by

EARL A. SURWIT, M.D.
5245 E. Knight
Tucson, Arizona 85712
U.S.A.

and

DAVID S. ALBERTS, M.D.
Section of Hematology and Oncology
Department of Internal Medicine
6th Floor Facility
The University of Arizona Health Sciences Ctr.
Tucson, Arizona 85724
U.S.A.

1987 **MARTINUS NIJHOFF PUBLISHERS**
a member of the KLUWER ACADEMIC PUBLISHERS GROUP
BOSTON / DORDRECHT / LANCASTER

Distributors

for the United States and Canada: Kluwer Academic Publishers, P.O. Box 358, Accord Station, Hingham, MA 02018-0358, USA
for the UK and Ireland: Kluwer Academic Publishers, MTP Press Limited, Falcon House, Queen Square, Lancaster LA1 1RN, UK
for all other countries: Kluwer Academic Publishers Group, Distribution Center, P.O. Box 322, 3300 AH Dordrecht, The Netherlands

Library of Congress Cataloging in Publication Data

Cervix cancer.

(Cancer treatment and research)
Includes index.
1. Cervix uteri--Cancer. I. Surwit, Earl A.
II. Alberts, David S. (David Samuel), 1939-
III. Series. [DNLM: 1. Cervix Neoplasms.
W1 CA693 / WP 480 C419]
RC280.U8C475 1986 616.99'466 86-17933
ISBN 0-89838-822-8

ISBN 0-89838-822-8 (this volume)
ISBN 90-247-2426-0 (series)

PRINTED IN THE NETHERLANDS

We would like to dedicate this book to our parents Jesse and Jeanine Surwit and Alfred and Esther Alberts Goldberg whose continued love, encouragement and support has lead to the success of our careers and the energy responsible for the completion of this book. Two sets of such special parents are rarely found in this complex world. Our hearts and best thoughts are with them always.

Table of Contents

Foreword to the series

Where do you begin to look for a recent, authoritative article on the diagnosis or management of a particular malignancy? The few general oncology textbooks are generally out of date. Single papers in specialized journals are informative but seldom comprehensive; these are more often preliminary reports on a very limited number of patients. Certain general journals frequently publish good indepth reviews of cancer topics, and published symposium lectures are often the best overviews available. Unfortunately, these reviews and supplements appear sporadically, and the reader can never be sure when a topic of special interest will be covered.

Cancer Treatment and Research is a series of authoritative volumes which aim to meet this need. It is an attempt to establish a critical mass of oncology literature covering virtually all oncology topics, revised frequently to keep the coverage up to date, easily available on a single library shelf or by a single personal subscription.

We have approached the problem in the following fashion. First, by dividing the oncology literature into specific subdivisions such as lung cancer, genitourinary cancer, pediatric oncology, etc. Second, by asking eminent authorities in each of these areas to edit a volume on the specific topic on an annual or biannual basis. Each topic and tumor type is covered in a volume appearing frequently and predictably, discussing current diagnosis, staging, markers, all forms of treatment modalities, basic biology, and more.

In *Cancer Treatment and Research,* we have an outstanding group of editors, each having made a major commitment to bring to this new series the very best literature in his or her field. Martinus Nijhoff Publishers has made an equally major commitment to the rapid publication of high quality books, and world-wide distribution.

Where can you go to find quickly a recent authoritative article on any major oncology problem? We hope that *Cancer Treatment and Research* provides an answer.

WILLIAM L. MCGUIRE
Series Editor

Preface

Cytological screening for the identification of intraepithelial neoplasia of the cervix as a precursor lesion for cervical cancer has been well established as an effective means for decreasing the incidence of invasive carcinoma. Despite these screening efforts, carcinoma of the cervix remains one of the more common malignancies in women and it is the leading cause of cancer death in many countries in the western hemisphere. It is estimated that in 1986 there will still be 14,000 new cases of invasive cancer, with 6,800 deaths in the United States alone. Unfortunately, many of these patients present with advanced disease, posing difficult management problems for the clinician responsible for their care.

The treatment of early stage invasive carcinoma of the cervix (lesions confined to the cervix and vagina) remains either radical surgery, radical radiation therapy or a combination thereof. This approach is extraordinarily effective in the vast majority of patients. However, there remains a subset of patients with early stage disease that are at high risk for recurrence.

Dr Kjorstad (Chapter 2) has identified adenocarcinomas and adenosquamous carcinomas as having a particularly poor prognosis. In addition, patients with more than three positive lymph nodes or with involvement of lymph nodes outside of the pelvis have a very poor prognosis. He has identified the CEA as a potentially predictive marker for these patients with poor prognosis, especially in patients with adenocarcinomas.

Dr Twiggs (Chapter 3) has identified the absence of progestational receptors in these tumors as a similar poor prognostic parameter to identify the high risk patient with early stage disease.

In advanced carcinoma of the cervix the problem is two-fold; that of controlling extensive pelvic disease and contending with the existence of extrapelvic disease outside of the usual pelvic radiation portals.

Dr Hacker (Chapter 4) very nicely elucidates the limitations of clinical staging in this setting and the applications of fine needle aspiration cytology for these patients. The technique of surgical staging is well described here;

however the primary problem, despite accurate surgical staging, still remains the control of bulky disease in the pelvis and secondarily, what therapy to offer those patients who are found to have extrapelvic disease. The addition of extended field radiation to the periaortic area has been associated with increased morbidity and, in most series, has not lead to a significant improvement in survival. As a consequence, we still need better control of pelvic disease in this patient population.

The problem of control of local disease with advanced carcinoma of the cervix may well be resolved by the addition of the transperineal template (irridium needle implant) for these patients, which is described extensively by Dr Aristizabel (Chapter 7). Previous attempts to solve the problem of local control by increasing dosages of external radiation therapy and/or the addition of radiation sensitizers have predominantly been unsuccessful and have lead to increasing rates of complications for these patients. Dr Aristizabel establishes quite clearly that the irridium needle implant can lead to an improvement of control of pelvic disease in advanced carcinoma of the cervix and more time will be required to establish that this will indeed translate into an improved survival for these patients.

Dr Piver (Chapter 8) presents very convincing data that hydroxyurea may well be an excellent radiosensitizer that could lead to an improvement in control of pelvic disease and translate into improved survival in these patients. These series are complicated by exclusion of patients with surgically proven extra-pelvic disease, and the variable of surgical staging in some of the studies. However, a recent Gynecologic Oncology Group study has confirmed Dr Piver's results.

The limitations of cytotoxic chemotherapy in carcinoma of the cervix are well delineated by Dr Thigpen (Chapter 9) in the discussion of single agent therapy and by Dr Brenner (Chapter 10) in the area of multiagent chemotherapy. A major problem in this field is that many patients, as noted above, fail in the pelvis after previous radiation therapy where there is fibrosis and very poor vasculature. As a consequence, it is very difficult to deliver adequate dosages of drugs to pelvic recurrences due to both poor vascular supply and impaired bone marrow from the radiation therapy. In addition, it may well be that resistent clones within the carcinoma of the cervix that are resistant to ionizing radiation may also be cross-resistant to cytotoxic drug therapy. Complete response rates in the treatment of carcinoma of the cervix have rarely been seen, and partial response rates that are seen rarely, if ever, lead to any meaningful improvement in survival for these patients. Unfortunately, no improvement in response rate and/or survival has yet been demonstrated in any multiagent chemotherapeutic regimen as compared to single agent therapy and, as might be predicted, increased toxicity is seen with the combination regimens. There does appear to be a rapid emergence of resistant clones in squamous cell carcinoma of the cervix, and it may well be that the best role for cytotoxic chemotherapy in this disease lies in earlier treatment for the high risk patient.

Unfortunately, the results to date of such neo-adjuvant chemotherapy in this setting of advanced disease have been disappointing, but the timing, sequencing and appropriate drugs to be selected may have yet to be determined in this area.

Dr Welander (Chapter 12) describes the potential application of the human tumor stem cell assay to help solve some of these problems. It is, in fact, in this area that this assay offers the most potential, rather than in the individualization of treatment planning for any given patient. The utilization of this system to identify potentially active new compounds and to define the optimal drug scheduling and concentration of these drugs, and to look at combinations of drugs could be a major help in solving the problems delineated above.

List of contributors

ALBERTS, David S., Section of Hematology and Oncology, Department of Medicine, Arizona Health Sciences Center, University of Arizona, 1501 N. Campbell, Tucson, AZ 85724, USA

ARISTIZABAL, Silvio A., Professor of Radiation Oncology, Department of Radiation Oncology, Arizona Health Sciences Center, University of Arizona, 1501 N. Campbell, Tucson, AZ 85724, USA

BEREK, Jonathan S., Associate Professor, UCLA School of Medicine, Division of Gynecologic Oncology, 10833 Le Conte Avenue, Los Angeles, CA 90024, USA

BRENNER, Dean E., Division of Oncology, Department of Medicine, Vanderbilt University, Nashville, TN 37232, USA

EINHORN, Nina, Department of Gynaecological Oncology, Karolinska sjukhuset, Radiumhemmet, 104 01 Stockholm, Sweden

HACKER, Neville F., Associate Professor, Director of Gynecologic Oncology, Department of Obstetrics and Gynecology, UCLA School of Medicine, Los Angeles, CA 90024, USA

KJORSTAD, Kjell E., The Norwegian Radium Hospital, Montebello, Oslo, Norway

LEUNG, Benjamin S., Professor, Director Division of Cell Biology and Reproduction, Department of Obstetrics and Gynecology, University of Minnesota Medical School, Minneapolis, MN 55455, USA

PARKER, JR., R. Lamar, Section on Gynecologic Oncology, Bowman Gray School of Medicine, 300 South Hawthorne Road, Winston-Salem, NC 27103, USA

PIVER, M. Steven, Associate Chief, Gynecology, Roswell Park Memorial Institute, University of Buffalo, Buffalo, NY 14203, USA

PODRATZ, Karl C., Assistant Professor of Obstetrics and Gynecology, Mayo Memorial Building, Mayo Clinic Foundation, 200 First Street, S.W., Rochester, MN 55905, USA

POTISH, Roger A., Associate Professor, Department of Therapeutic Radiology, Box 395, Mayo Memorial Building, Minneapolis, MN 55455, USA

SURWIT, Earl A., Gynecologic Oncology, 5245 E. Knight, Tucson, AZ 85712, USA

SYMMONDS, Richard E., Professor and Chairman Emeritus, Gynecologic and General Surgery, Mayo Clinic, Mayo Graduate School, Rochester, MN 55901, USA

THIGPEN, J. Tate, University of Mississippi, School of Medicine, 2500 North State Street, Jackson, MS 39216, USA

TWIGGS, Leo B., Associate Professor, Director of Gynecologic Oncology, Department of Obstetrics and Gynecology, Box 395, Mayo Memorial Building, Minneapolis, MN 55455, USA

WEINER, Sheldon A., Assistant Professor, Department of Obstetrics and Gynecology, College of Medicine and the Arizona Cancer Center, University of Arizona, 1501 N. Campbell, Tucson, AZ 85724, USA

WELANDER, Charles E., Section on Gynecologic Oncology, Bowman Gray School of Medicine, 300 South Hawthorne Road, Winston-Salem, NC 27103, USA

1. Cervical dysplasia

SHELDON A. WEINER

Introduction

Few malignancies lend themselves as well to early diagnosis as does cervical cancer, and the intent of this chapter will be to discuss recent advances in the understanding of the pathogenesis of cervical preneoplasia, its diagnosis, treatment, and possible prevention.

Etiology

Epidemiologic evidence

The epidemiologic evidence linking early sexual activity and promiscuity with the development of cervical dysplasia has led to the widespread acceptance of the belief that this is a sexually transmitted disease [1–3]. What still remains to be determined is the identification of the etiologic agent. In the 1970s, attention focused on the herpes simplex type II virus, however, 15 years of follow-up have failed to yield the definitive evidence of it being the etiologic agent [4]. Although this agent is not entirely discarded, current research is focusing on the role of the human papilloma virus (HPV) in cervical neoplasia. A recent epidemologic evaluation of the association of a variety of sexually transmitted diseases with abnormal cervical cytology revealed a relative risk of six for HPV vs. 0.8 for herpes infection [5]. While the role of sexual activity in the transmission of HPV is well established [6], the possibility that the male may serve as a vector for the transmission of cervical carcinoma is not as well studied. Evidence that supports this hypothesis is the reported increased association of cervical cancer in wives of men with penile cancer [7, 8]. Similarly, Kessler has shown a higher incidence of cervical cancer being seen among women married to men whose previous wives had cervical carcinoma [9]. Levine has reported that 53% of

E.A. Surwit, D.S. Alberts (eds) Cervix Cancer.
 ISBN 0-89838-822-8. Printed in the Netherlands.

male partners of a select group of women with CIN had detectable penile condyloma [10], and HPV DNA has been recovered in human ejaculate [11]. Reid and associates have shown that histologic evidence of HPV is seven times more likely in women with dysplasia or invasive carcinoma of the cervix when compared to a matched set of controls [12]. The mean age of women with condyloma is lower than that of women with HPV infection and CIN [13], suggesting that HPV infection may precede the development of CIN. Similarly, patients with CIN alone tend to be older than patients with HPV and CIN, which suggests either HPV may initiate CIN, or alternatively, may accelerate the neoplastic transformation [14].

Histologic evidence

In an attempt to evaluate objectively whether or not HPV infection was morphologically distinct from CIN, Reid and associates developed a semi-objective scoring system to evaluate 24 different histologic criteria in the interpretation of 72 targeted biopsies. They concluded that HPV infection lay along a morphologic continuum with CIN, and that differences between groups were more a matter of degree rather than representative of separate entities [15].

The presence of papillomaviral capsid antigen has been detected in milder forms of cervical dysplasia [16–18], however proof of HPV infection in the more severely dysplastic, aneuploid cells had been lacking, due to the inability of transformed, premalignant cells to express viral specific proteins [19]. With the recent development of type specific HPV DNA probes, a number of investigators have been able to demonstrate the presence of viral DNA in a variety of cervical dysplasias and carcinomas [20, 21]. It appears that types 6 and 11 are more often seen with the milder forms of dysplasia, while types 16 and 18 tend to be found more commonly in cervical carcinomas [22, 23].

Animal models, human models

The inability to grow HPV *in vitro* has limited studies of its oncogenic potential. However, papilloma virus infection of the domestic rabbit by the Shope virus produces warty lesions which become malignant in 25% of cases [24]. Similarly, bovine papilloma virus has caused transformation of tissue culture cells, as well as inducing intestinal and bladder malignancies in cattle [25]. Occasional malignant conversion of human vulvar condylomas, laryngeal papillomas and skin warts has been documented [21].

Diagnosis

The advent of cytologic screening by Papanicolau revolutionized the early detection of cervical neoplasia. Subsequently, the acceptance of the colposcope over the past decade has added another tool to the armamentarium of the gynecologist-pathologist. Currently, in the hands of a well-trained colposcopist, accurate histologic diagnosis can be arrived at with essentially no morbidity in over 90% of cases [26]. The dilemma currently facing the clinician is to decide which patients with dysplasia need to be treated, and which patients can be conservatively followed. The current trend is to treat all women with CIN, since we are currently unable to predict, on an individual basis, who will experience malignant progression of her disease. Two recent developments may allow us to alter this 'shotgun' approach.

DNA spectrophotometry

Recent work by Yao S. Fu has shown a strong correlation between DNA ploidy patterns and the subsequent outcome of untreated cervical preneoplasia. In 120 women studied, 89% of patients with diploid or polyploid lesions had spontaneous regression, whereas 80% of patients with aneuploid lesions had persistence of their disease. No patients with diploid or polyploid lesions progressed to cancer, while 11% of patients with aneuploid lesions developed cervical carcinoma [27].

Currently, this technology is expensive and not widely available, but ultimately, this may assist clinicians in deciding which patients are unlikely to have spontaneous regression of their lesion.

In situ *DNA hybridization*

The discovery that certain HPV subtypes are more commonly found in association with higher degrees of cervical dysplasia implies that we may someday be able to target treatment towards those patients infected with the 'oncogenic' virus. Current methodology using Southern blot hybridization with known DNA probes is not widely applicable as a screening modality. Recently, Wagner *et al.* have reported on an *in situ* hybridization technique on cervical swabs taken for routine screening [28]. Of 22 cases of CIN III, 15 hybridized with types 16 and 18, four hybridized with type 11, and three were negative. In 13 cases of mild or moderate dysplasia, only four reacted with types 16 or 18, four reacted with type 11, and three were negative.

While these new technologies present exciting new possibilities in the management of cervical dysplasia, one must proceed cautiously until the true meaning of the information being generated is better understood. It is noteworthy that although some of the data suggests there may be two patient populations, if one looks closely, it becomes apparent that there is some degree of overlap between the benign end of the spectrum with those patients who are felt to have a malignant precursor. Some patients with CIN III are infected with type 11 HPV; does this mean that these lesions can be ignored? Similarly, there is overlap between DNA ploidy patterns and histologic evidence of pre-malignancy. Reid reported on five out of 17 polyploid lesions which contained abnormal mitotic figures [29], a finding not consistent with the spectrophotometric prediction of the benign nature of these lesions. Until we are better able to understand the prognostic significance of these new diagnostic modalities, the clinician must continue to treat all dysplasias as potentially pre-malignant.

Treatment

Although the clinician must treat all dysplasias as potentially premalignant, it is widely recognized that spontaneous regression may occur, and progression to invasive carcinoma is not a foregone conclusion. The dilemma for the clinician, however, is that no accurate information exists regarding spontaneous progression and regression rates. Because of the inability to predict the natural history of cervical dysplasia in a given patient, most clinicians elect to treat all CIN.

Current treatment modalities for CIN are highly successful and consist of local destruction or excision of the transformation zone. The three major methods of local ablation are cryotherapy, laser and electrocoagulation. Table 1 lists several recent series utilizing the different methodologies, and as one can see, cure rates are in the range of 85–90% for all these techniques. Notably, cure rates tended to be lower in those series where an ECC was not performed.

In this country, cryotherapy is the most widely utilized technique. Failure rates of almost 50% have been noted when a single, 3-min freeze has been utilized [30, 31], whereas a double freeze technique is reported to lower failure rates to 18.7% [32]. Persistent lesions can be retreated, resulting in greater than 95% cures in a recent series by Creasman *et al.* [32]. Fertility rates and pregnancy outcome do not appear to be adversely affected by this treatment modality [30, 33].

Laser vaporization of the transformation zone is increasingly becoming a preferred treatment modality by many investigators. As can be seen in Table 1, cure rates between the two methods appear similar. In three prospective randomized trials comparing cryosurgery with laser, similar cure rates were observed in all series [34–36]. Jobson did report that healing was

Table 1. Destruction techniques in the treatment of CIN.

	Success rates after one treatment (repeated treatment)					
Method/author	ECC	N	CIN I	CIN II	CIN III	Total
Electrocoagulation						
Peckham *et al.*	(+)	110	94	88	84	89
Jonassen and Bergstrom	+	100		not stated		82
Schuurmans and Carmichael	(+)	426	90	82	87	86
Cryocoagulation						
Einerth	+	59		not stated		92 [95]
Ostergard	+	344	94	93	80	92
Kristensen and Hansen	(+)	125	–	89	88	88 [93]
Charles *et al.*	–	130	82	83	82	82
Wright and Davies	+	152	93	88	75	86
Peckham *et al.*	(+)	247	97	94	87	94
Townsend and Richart	+	100	100	95	91	93
Hemmingson and Stenson	+	105	91*		85	88
van Lent *et al.*	(+)	102	–	–	93	93
Creasman *et al.*	+	770	95	93	82	90 [96]
Arof *et al.*	(+)	265	92	82	73	85
Bryson *et al.*	(+)	422	–	–	93	93
Laser evaporation (3 mm)						
Jordan	–	210	92	100	88	92
Benedet *et al.*	–	179	100	87	78	82
Wright and Davies	+	131	100	98	92	97
Bellina *et al.*	–	256	99	92	86	93
Anderson	–	441	89	80	74	76 [98]
Burke	+	131	84	86	78	82 [87]
Townsend and Richard	+	100	90	92	87	89
Wright *et al.*	–	429	98	95	95	95 [100]
Popkin	+	138	89	92	90	91
Evansand Monaghan	–	410		not stated		93 [96]
Baggish	+	414	94	90	91	92 [96]
Berget (unpublished results)	+	71	100	98	100	99 [100]

+ Indicates that ECC has been performed in all cases in the study; (+) indicates that ECC has been performed in selected cases in the study; and – indicates that ECC has not been performed; * indicates combined success rate of CIN I and II.
([39], reprinted with permission).

better after laser ablation, as 86% of patients had satisfactory colposcopy on follow-up vs. only 53% of those patients treated with cryotherapy. Those investigators that prefer laser vaporization over cryosurgery site better preservation of the squamo-columnar junction, and better depth control as advantages of this technique. As with cryosurgery, laser does not appear to adversely affect pregnancy outcome [37].

Methods of surgical excision include conization or hysterectomy. In general, there are negligible differences in recurrence rates of CIN when either modality is used. Kolstad and Klem reported on 1121 cases of CIS and observed a 2.4% recurrence rate when conization was used vs. 1.2% when a hysterectomy was performed [38]. Berget, in reviewing the literature on this subject, concluded that while the recurrence rates are slightly higher with conization, 3% vs. 0.8% for CIN, and 0.6% vs. 0.3% for carcinoma, the difference did not justify favoring hysterectomy over conization [39]. One should utilize the more definitive surgical procedure only if there are coexisting conditions which would make hysterectomy preferable. Similarly, involvement of the margins of the conization does not necessitate immediate hysterectomy. In Kolstad's series, 21 of 25 patients with CIS at the surgical margins were recurrence free from 5–15 years after the surgical procedure. If preservation of fertility is desired, a period of close observation is warranted.

Prevention

Background in chemoprevention

Clearly, the most significant impact that can be made on cancer mortality is in the realm of prevention. Three major areas exist towards which intervention can be directed. Primary prevention consists of preventing exposure to known carcinogens. Examples would include abstinence from tobacco or eliminating asbestos from the work place. Efforts in this area obviously need to be directed toward social and political change. Secondary prevention involves modulating the initiation or promotion phase of carcinogenesis using various biologic response modifiers. This can involve the use of antioxidants (vitamin E, butylated hydroxytoluene, etc.) to quench free radicals, thereby functioning as antiinitiators in preventing cell damage. Alternatively, antipromoters (retinoids, proteases, steroids) can be used to prevent the phenotypic expression of malignancy in the transformed cell. The cervical epithelial cell infected with human papilloma virus is an example of the latter. Finally, tertiary prevention involves the treatment of established preneoplasia, and the previously mentioned techniques of laser vaporization or cryosurgery represent this type of approach.

Biologic response modifiers

Currently, there are two major compounds which have undergone limited clinical trials in the treatment of CIN, retinoids and interferons. Although the specific mechanisms remain unclear, numerous animal studies have confirmed the role of retinoid compounds as enhancers of both cellular and humoral immunity [40]. In murine systems, the cytoxicity of killer T cells and stimulated macrophages to tumor cells was augmented using retinoic acid [40]. Enhancement of graft rejection using either retinoic acid or retinyl palmitate has also been noted in mouse models [40]. Humoral response in mice has been shown to be enhanced when retinol, retinal or retinoic acid was administered prior to an immunologic challenge with bovine gamma globulin [40]. The exact role that immunomodulation plays in human systems remains to be determined.

However, retinoids have long been know to be modulators of cellular differentiation. As early as 1965 Chu and Malmgren demonstrated that 10% vitamin A palmitate was able to prevent the induction of cervical carcinomas initiated by 10% DMBA in Syrian hamsters [41]. Numerous other animal models have confirmed the ability of retinoids to function as antipromoters. Not only are these compounds capable of preventing malignant transformation, but they have been shown capable of altering established malignant cell lines. This has been demonstrated in embryonal cell carcinoma, melanoma, promyelocytic leukemia, breast carcinoma and cervical carcinoma, to name a few [42, 43]. Therefore, it is a logical extension of this concept to attempt to use retinoids clinically to prevent the phenotypic expression of neoplasia induced by papilloma virus, as well as to reverse established preneoplasia.

At the University of Arizona we have acquired extensive experience with preliminary trials utilizing topically applied transretinoic acid (TRA) in patients with CIN [44, 45]. Of 56 patients treated in phase I and phase II trials, 22 (39%) had a CR. When dose response effect was assessed, 20/42 (47.6%) patients treated with high dose TRA experienced a CR vs. 2/14 patients (14%) treated with low dose TRA. Responses were seen in all grades of dysplasia. A randomized phase III trial comparing placebo vs. TRA is currently in progress.

There are some preliminary reports of activity of interferons (INF) in treating CIN. Nine of 11 patients with CIN treated at the University of Hong Kong [46], and seven of 14 patients with vaginal intra epithelial neoplasia or CIN treated at the Instituto Nazionale Tumori in Italy [47], experienced a CR after intralesional injection of INF. Moller has reported on six patients treated with INF applied via a cervical cap, three of whom had a CR and three of whom had improvement [48]. In patients treated with intralesional injection, systemic toxicity was noted and this will probably preclude this route of administration in future trials of INF in CIN. Topically applied INF is apparently without toxicity and the results of future trials utilizing this modality are eagerly awaited. Not only does interferon offer the potential for immunomodulation, as do retinoids, but it is also a well known antiviral agent, a useful adjunct in a disease that is felt to be virally mediated.

Conclusion

New diagnostic modalities offer potential insight into the pathogenesis of CIN, as well as the possibility of more selective therapeutic intervention. Until that time, the mainstay of treatment of cervical preneoplasia continues to be cytologic screening followed by biopsy and transformation zone ablation. Given the relative ease with which this can be accomplished, it continues to be somewhat discouraging that so many patients continue to elude attempts at tertiary prevention. New trials utilizing biologic response modifers for secondary chemoprevention may offer future clinicians the opportunity to target a high risk population for intervention, with the ultimate hope of preventing the phenotypic expression of cervical neoplasia.

Acknowledgement

The author wishes to acknowledge the assistance of Christi Wagner in the preparation of this manuscript.

References

1. Kessler II. 1976. Human cervical Cancer as a veneral disease. Cancer Res 36:783.
2. Rotkin ID. 1973. A comparison review of key epidemiological studies in cervical cancer related to current searches for transmissable agents. Cancer Res 33:1353–1367.
3. Thomas DB. 1973. An epidemiologic study of carcinoma in situ and squamous dysplasia of the uterine cervix. Am J Epidemiol 98:10–28.
4. Nahmias AJ, Sacoanabor S. 1978. The genital herpes – cervical cancer hypothesis – 10 years later. prog Exp Tumor Res 21:117–139.
5. Franceschi S, Doll R, Gallway J *et al.* 1983. Genital warts and cervical neoplasia: An epidemiological study. Br J Cancer 48:621.
6. Oriel JD. 1971. Natural history of genital warts. Br J Vener Dis 47:1–13.
7. Graham S, Priore R, Graham M, Browne R, Burnett W, West D. 1979. Genital Cancer in wives of penile cancer patients. Cancer 44:1970–1974.
8. Smith PG, Kinlen LJ, White GC, Adelstein AM, Fox AJ. 1980. Mortality of wives of men dying with cancer of the penis. Br J Cancer 41:422–428.
9. Kessler II. 1974. Cervical cancer, epidemiology in historical perspective. J Reprod Med 12:173.
10. Levine RU, Crum CP, Herman E, Silvers D, Ferenczy A, Richart R. 1984. Cervical papillomavirus infection and intraepithelial neoplasia: a study of male sexual partners. Obstet Gynecol 64:16–20.

11. Ostrow RS. 1984. Veneral Transmission of Human Papilloma Viruses; The Presence of HPV DNA in Human Ejaculate. Human Papilloma Virus and Squamous Carcinoma Conference Chicago, Illinois, Oct 1984.
12. Reid R, Stanhope CR, Herschman BR, Booth E, Phibbs GD, Smith JP. 1982. Genital warts and cervical cancer. I. Evidence of an association between subclinical papillovmavirus infection and cervical malignancy. Cancer 50:377–387.
13. Mazur MT, Cloud GA. 1984. The koilocyte and cervical intraepithelial neoplasia: time-trend analysis of a recent decade. Am J Obstet Gynecol 150:354–358.
14. Woodruff JD, Braun L, Cavaliere R *et al.* 1980. Immunological identification of papillomavirus antigen in paraffin-processed condyloma tissues from the female genital tract. Obstet Gynecol 56:727.
15. Reid R, Crum CP, Herschman Br, Fu YS, Braun L, Shah KV, Agronow SJ, Stanhope CR. 1984. Genital warts and cervical cancer. Ill. Subclinical papillomaviral infection and cervical neoplasia are linked by a spectrum of continuous morphologic and biologic change. Cancer 53:943–953.
16. Crum CP, Egawa K, Barron B, Fenoglio CM, Levine RU, Richart RM. 1983. Human papillomavirus infection (condyloma) of the cervix and cervical intraepithelial neoplasia: a histopathologic and statistical analysis. Gynecol Oncol 15:88.
17. Ferenczy A, Braun L, Shah KV. 1981. Human papillomavirus (HPV) in condylomatous lesions of the cervix. Am J Surg Pathol 5:661.
18. Kurman RJ, Sanz LE, Jenson AB *et al.* 1982. Papillomavirus infection of the cervix. I. Correlation of histology with viral structural antigens and DNA sequences. Int J Gynecol Path I:17.
19. Meyer G. 1978. Polyoma virus, as a model for viral skin carcinogenesis. Bull Cancer 65:145.
20. Durst M, Gissman L, Ikenberg H, Zur Hausen H. 1983. A new type of papillomaviral DNA from a cervical carcinoma and its prevalence in cancer biopsies from different geographic regions. Proc Natl Acad Sci 80:3812.
21. Zur Hausen H. 1977. Human papillomaviruses and their possible role in squamous cell carcinomas. Curr Top Microbiol Immunol 78:1.
22. Richart RM, Ferenczy A, Meisels A, Syrjanen K, Zur Hausen H. 1984. Condyloma virus and cervical cancer - How strong a link? Contemp. Ob Gyn 23:210–224.
23. Crum CP, Ikenberg H, Richart RM, Gissman L. 1984. Human papillomavirus type 16 and early cervical neoplasia. N Engl J Med 310:880–883.
24. Syverton JT. 1952. The pathogenesis of the rabitt papilloma-to-carcinoma sequence. Ann NY Acad Sci 54:1126.
25. Jarrett WFH, McNeil PE, Zaird HM *et al.* 1980. Papillomaviruses in benign and malignant tumors of cattle. Cold Spring Harbor Conf Cell Proliferation 7:215.
26. Stafl A, Mattingly RF. 1973. Colposcopic diagnosis of cervical neoplasia. Obstet Gynecol 41:168–176.
27. Fu YS. 1984. Differing DNA patterns in CN. Human Papilloma Virus and Squamous Carcinoma Conference, Chicago, Illinois, Oct, 1984.
28. Wagner D, Ikenberg H, Boehm N, Gissmann L. 1984. Identification of human papillomavirus in cervical swabs by deoxyribonucleic acid in situ hybridization. Obstet. Gynecol 64:767–772.
29. Reid R, Fu YS, Herschman Br, Crum CP, Braun L, Shah KV, Agronow SJ, Stanhope CR. 1984. Genital warts and cervical cancer, CI. The relationship between aneuploid and polyploid cervical lesions. Am J Obstet Gynecol 150:190–199.
30. Charles EH, Savage EW. 1980. Cryosurgical treatment of cervical intraepithelial neoplasia. Obstet Gynecol Survey 35:539–548.
31. Creasman WT, Weed JC Jr, Curry SL *et al.* 1973. Efficacy of cryosurgical treatment of severe cervical intraepithelial neoplasia. Obstet Gynecol 41:501.

32. Creasman WT, Hinshaw WM, Clarke-Pearson DL. 1984. Cryosurgery in the management of cervical intraepithelial neoplasia. Obstet Gynecol 63:145–149.
33. Weed JC, Curry SL, Duncan ID, Parker RT, Creasman WT. 1978. Fertility after cryosurgery of the cervix. Obstet Gynecol 52:245.
34. Townsend DE, Richart RM. 1983. Cryotherapy and carbon dioxide laser management of cervical intraepithelial neoplasia: a controlled comparison. Cryotherapy vs. CO_2 Laser in CIN 61:75–78.
35. Jobson VW, Homesley HD. 1984. Comparison of cryosurgery and carbon dioxide laser ablation for treatment of cervical intraepithelial neoplasia. Colpo Gynecol Laser Surg 1:173–180.
36. Kerivan PH, Smith IR, Naltalin NJ. 1985. A study of cryosurgery and the CO_2 laser in treatment of carcinoma in situ (Cin III) of the uterine cervix. Gynecol Oncol 22:195–200.
37. Anderson MC, Horwell DH, Broby Z. 1984. Outcome of pregnancy after laser vaporization conization. Colpo Gynecol Laser Surg 1:35–37.
38. Kolstad P, Klem V. 1976. Long-term follow-up of 1121 cases of carcinoma in situ. Obstet Gynecol 48:125–129.
39. Berget A, Lenstrup C. 1985. Cervical intraepithelial neoplasia. Examination, treatment and follow-up. Obstet Gynecol Survey 40:545–552.
40. Lotan R. 1980. Effects of vitamin A and its analogues (retinoids) in normal and neoplastic cells. Biochem Biophys Acta 605:33.
41. Chu, EW, Malmgren RA. 1965. An inhibitory effect of vitamin A on the induction of tumors of forestomach and cervix in the Syrian hamster by carcinogenic polycyclic hydrocarbons. Cancer Res 25:884–885.
42. Peck GL. 1981. Chemoprevention of cancer with retinoids. Gynecol Oncol 12:5331.
43. Meyskens FL. 1981. Modulation of abnormal growth by retinoids: a clinical perspective of the biological phenomenon. Life Sci 28:2323–2327.
44. Surwit EA, Graham V, Droegemueller W, Alberts D, Chvapil M, Door R, Davis JR, Meyskens FL. 1982. Evaluation of topically applied trans-retinoic acid in the treatment of cervical intraepithelial lesions. Am J Ob Gyn 143:821–823.
45. Weiner SA, Meyskens FL Jr, Surwit EA, Alberts DS, Levine NS. 1985. Response of human papilloma-associated diseases to retinoids (vitamin A derivatives) papilloma viruses: Molecular and Clinical Aspects, UCLA Volume 32 (in press).
46. Oncology News, July-August 1984, p 4.
47. Stefanon B, DePalo G, Rilke F, Pilotti S, Ghione M. 1984. Human fibroblast interferon (HFI) in cervical and vulvar intraepithelial neoplasia with viral cytopathic effect (VCE). American Society in Colposcopy and Cervical Pathology and Gynecologic Laser Society, Lake Buena Vista, FL, March, 1984 (Abst #45).
48. Moeller BR, Johannesen P, Osther K, Ulmsteen U, Hastrup J, Berg K. 1983. Treatment of dysplasia of the cervical epithelium with an interferon gel. Obstet Gynecol 62:625–629.

2. The management of the high risk patient with early invasive carcinoma of the cervix

KJELL E. KJORSTAD

Introduction

Treatment results in early stages of cancer of the cervix are favourable with 5-year survival rates up to 100% if the tumor is limited in its volume and depth of infiltration. Dissemination occurs relatively late and predominantly by the lymphatic system. Even widespread local, or regional disease can be cured.

If a truly localized lesion exists, its treatment should be simple and the results excellent. The FIGO staging system recognizes a subgroup of stage I, but does not clearly define this lesion. In most centers the depth of tumor infiltration into the stroma is used to delineate a tumor with metastatic potential from one with a high probability of dissemination, but there is no general agreement on how this minimal lesion, usually designated as stage IA, should be defined. The most commonly used criterion is probably an infiltration depth of less than 5 mm into the stroma. With current therapeutic methods, between 95 and 99% of these patients will be alive 5 years after treatment. However, some of them eventually succumb to regional or distant recurrences, showing that so called 'minimal disease' can in fact be disseminated. With increasing local tumor volume the probability of dissemination also increases. Therefore excellent average survival figures for the individual stages are no guarantee for an optimal prognosis in the individual case. High risk patients can be recognized within each stage or within a subgroup of a stage. For example, patients in clinical stage I are usually reported to have a 5-year survival between 80% and 90%, but if metastases in the common iliac lymph nodes are found in stage I, the survival chances are almost none.

E.A. Surwit, D.S. Alberts (eds) Cervix Cancer.
 ISBN 0-89838-822-8. Printed in the Netherlands.

Definition of the high risk patient

A high risk patient may be defined as one with a suboptimal prognosis in relation to the average results achieved in the corresponding stage. Obviously we are dealing with two main problems: (1) failure within the treatment area with local or regional recurrence or, (2) unrecognized dissemination with relapses in untreated areas of the body.

Treatment and definition of early lesions

There is considerable disagreement between radiotherapists and surgeons concerning the optimal treatment for patients with early stage disease, but there is no room for the fruitless discussion on the superiority of one treatment modality over the other. In early disease (stages I and IIA) radiotherapy and surgery are both effective. Treatment reports are often biased by the preference of the investigator for one specific treatment modality. The fact that some patients are unsuited for surgery is evident. Equally evident is the fact that surgery in some instances is the method of choice. It is in the patient's best interest that she should have her case judged by therapists who are able to evaluate her entire situation and who feel free to recommend the best available therapy. Selection of the proper treatment modality is probably the best insurance for an optimal result.

Methods

Prospective, randomized trials are urgently needed, but extremely difficult to accomplish. Results and complication rates from one institution cannot uncritically be compared with those from another, as personal skill and experience with one method will vary. Valid conclusions, however, can be reached by analyses of materials sampled in one institution if the number of cases is large enough, and the principles of treatment are not changed during the sampling period. The following discussion is a presentation based on experience from one institution, the Norwegian Radium Hospital. All three main treatment modalities are used in our clinic and performed by the same physicians. Our clinical series are large and hopefully without bias. The follow-up is complete.

Prognostic features

A number of factors of prognostic significance can be recognized in cervical cancer patients. Some of these factors are extremely important and will to a large extent determine the fate of the patient. Others are of more legendary interest and their significance is not established. The understanding and recognition of these factors may help in the interpretation of the total situation of the patient and can also be helpful in the planning of treatment. The prognostic impact of age, tumor type, differentiation, vessel invasion, radiosensitivity and disseminated disease has been systematically studied in our clinic. A summary of our findings is presented under the present heading.

Age

Cancer of the cervix is a rare disease in very young women. In many countries there has been a marked increase in the incidence of severe dysplasia and carcinoma *in situ* since the introduction of large scale cytology, and younger women represent a substantial proportion of this increase. In Norway, there has also been an apparent increase in the incidence of invasive lesions for patients under the age of 35, especially during the last 10–15 years (Figure 1).

Treatment results for young women have been reported to be worse, equal or better than the total cervical cancer population [1–5], but the prevailing opinion is that the prognosis for young women is worse than the average. There are two large studies by Truelsen [1] and Lindell [2] which conclude that cancer of the cervix is a particularly malignant disease in young women. Most patients in these reports had been treated with radiotherapy

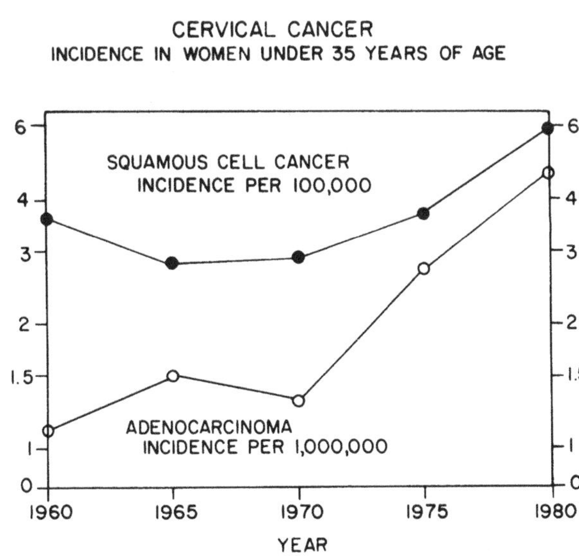

Figure 1. Incidence of cervical cancer in Norway, 1960–1980.

alone, and it was concluded that young women had a higher incidence of special kinds of tumors characterized among other features by a reduced radiosensitivity. This view was supported by Kottmeier [3], who stated that young women with cancer of the cervix should be treated by surgery rather than radiotherapy.

In our own experience [5] no difference could be found in treatment results in 139 patients younger than 35 years of age compared with the total number of 2002 patients treated in the same time period (Table 1).

In conclusion, studies of the literature do not clearly substantiate that young age itself is a negative prognostic factor. It may well be, however, that younger age groups have a larger relative proportion of tumor types with prognostically unfavourable features than cervical cancer populations in general.

Tumor type

Adenocarcinoma accounts for 5–10% of all cervical tumors. Therefore large published series of treatment results are infrequent. Some authors believe that adenocarcinomas are less radiosensitive than squamous cell cancers, and many reports confirm the inferior treatment results achieved by radiotherapy in patients with adenocarcinomas. It has also been postulated that adenocarcinomas of early stages have a higher metastatic potential than squamous cell cancers.

A study from the Radium Hospital [6] showed that patients with adenocarcinomas treated with radiotherapy only, had an inferior prognosis compared with patients with squamous cell cancers in corresponding stages. In stage I no difference in prognosis could be found between patients with adenocarcinomas and squamous cell cancers, provided the therapy included surgery of the primary tumor, with or without preoperative intracavitary treatment (Tables 2 and 3). In a report on the metastatic potential of ade-

Table 1. Survival rates for 139 patients under 35 years of age compared with the total cervical cancer population.

		5-year survival (%)	
	No. of patients	18–34	Total
Stages I and II A	1310	83	82
Stages II B–IV	692	35	39
Total	2002		

nocarcinomas [7], no difference could be found between different tumor types.

We conclude that the cure rates for the total group of patients with adenocarcinomas are clearly inferior to that of patients with squamous cell carcinoma and that radiotherapy is less effective in these patients. The histologic diagnosis of an adenocarcinoma is therefore a prognostic factor of significant importance that should influence the choice of treatment and include surgery, if possible.

Tumor differentiation

The prognostic impact of tumor differentiation is another issue under debate. Beecham [8], in a report from the Radium Hospital, was unable to correlate tumor grade with prognosis for squamous cell carcinomas. Differentiation alone is not sufficient to classify squamous cell carcinomas into tumors with a low or high potential malignancy. Stendahl [9] has shown that several intercorrelated histologic features need to be examined if morphologic criteria are to be of prognostic value.

Completely undifferentiated tumors as well as small cell types and tumors with endocrine activity ('apudomas'), are highly malignant. These tu-

Table 2. Five-year survival for 102 patients with adenocarcinoma compared with 1900 patients with squamous cell carcinoma.

	Adenocarcinoma		Squamous cell carcinoma	
Stage	No.	% survival	No.	% survival
I	47	83 [a]	892	87 [a]
II	32	34	713	63
III	14	14	210	28
IV	9	0	85	4
Total	102	51 [b]	1900	68 [b]

[a] Difference not significant.
[b] Difference highly significant.

Table 3. Five-year survival for patients with adenocarcinoma in stages I B and II A in relation to treatment.

	No. of patients	% survival
Operated	50	82
Radiotherapy only	15	40

mors are very radiosensitive, and primary results in early stages after irradiation may look promising. Local recurrence and metastases are, however, the rule and conventional therapy seems to be quite inadequate. Fortunately these types are very rare, but might become more prevalent as the incidence of conventional types of cervical cancer is decreasing. Little is known about the optimal treatment of these tumor types, except that chemotherapy seems to be indicated in addition to irradiation or surgery.

Vessel invasion

Destruction and infiltration are basic properties of malignant tissues and linked to the mestastic potential of a tumor. In order to reach distant parts of the body the cancer cells must enter lymphatic channels or blood vessels. Such invasion is probably always present, but our possibility to observe this phenomenon is proportional to the amount of tissue subjected to microscopic examination. The important question is whether observed vessel invasion has a prognostic significance of its own. Roche [10] observed lymphatic involvement in 57% of 30 cases of microinvasive carcinoma and concluded that it was of no prognostic value. On the other hand Larsson [11] found unquestionable vascular involvement in 8.5% of 343 patients of all stages and concluded that it had a prognostic impact more important than the depth of infiltration. The experience of the Radium Hospital [12] confirms the prognostic importance of vessel invasion. In 122 patients with microinvasive carcinoma, unquestionable vessel invasion was found in eight (6.6%) and the disease recurred in five. Metastases in the pelvic lymph nodes were found in five patients and three of them had observable lymphatic vessel invasion.

Radiosensitivity

Radiotherapy has been the cornerstone of treatment for cervical cancer since the beginning of this century. Due to the extreme radiotolerance of the normal uterus and vagina, tumoricidal doses can almost always be given to the cervix by means of intracavitary implants of isotopes without serious damage to the normal tissues. This accounts for the very high primary healing rate after brachytherapy. In clinical stage I, 98% of squamous cell cancers are primarely cured after local irradiation, and recurrence at the primary site is seen in only 5%. Theoretically radioresistance should be of importance only in patients treated with radiotherapy, but we have repeatedly shown that radioresistant squamous cell tumors of the cervix have a high frequency of metastases as well as a high recurrence rate, even in

patients treated by surgery. Our ability to recognize radioresistant tumors prior to treatment is very limited. Observations in our department have indicated that these tumors might be different from other cervical tumors in several biological aspects. One of the more interesting features is that subnormal amounts of Carcinoembryonic antigen are released from such tumors [13].

The effect on prognosis of residual tumor in the hysterectomy specimen after preoperative intracavitary irradiation is shown in Table 4. When surgery is performed 6 weeks after radium insertions, a number of tumors will still not be primarely healed. All these cases cannot be designated as radioresistant, as the tumor tissue may not be viable, but the true radioresistant tumors will be found among patients with residual tumors. It is important to realize that residual tumor in a hysterectomy specimen is not a function of the size of the primary tumor only, and that this observation has a prognostic significance of its own.

Dissemination

Despite the clinical impression of limited disease, some patients have widespread dissemination at the time of diagnosis. At least 10% of patients in stages IB and IIA have disease beyond the pelvis. These patients cannot be cured by local or regional treatment and with conventional diagnostic procedures, we are unable to identify them.

Lymphatic spread is by far the most important mode of dissemination in early stages. Within the pelvis, the primary and secondary lymph nodes have been studied and defined by Henriksen [14]. The concept that cancer of the cervix spreads along reasonably fixed routes from primary to secondary group of nodes has been widely accepted. The gloomy prognostic outlook if spread has reached the secondary nodes (pre-sacral and common iliac groups) is well known.

Spread within the pelvis is obvious in operated patients and most centers recognize the high risk status of such patients and give postoperative radio-

Table 4. Recurrence in relation to residual tumor found in hysterectomy specimens patients with stage I B cancer of the cervix treated with preoperative radium.

Site of recurrence	Residual tumor % of total	No residual tumor % of total
Central & pelvic	27.3	7.8
Distant	15.9	5.2
Total	43.2	12.9

therapy. Whether the added radiotherapy is really indicated and enhances the chances of cure, is obscure [15]. The prognostic importance of pelvic lymph node dissemination is pronounced as 50% of these patients will die from their disease, but the extent of the dissemination and the localization of the metastases are of paramount importance. The reported incidence of pelvic lymph node mestastasis in operable patients varies from 10 to 30%. The reason for this is that different selective criteria are used in different centers. If radiotherapy is the only treatment, pelvic dissemination is usually undiscovered. Therefore comparison between the over-all results achieved by radiotherapy and surgery can only be done in unselected patient materials. In a publication from the Radium Hospital [16] it was shown that radiotherapy is as efficient as surgery in every respect, and that over-all complication rates are the same for both procedures.

Many years of experience with radiotherapy has shown that this method is stretched to the maximum of its efficacy. Higher doses, locally by intracavitary implants, or regionally by external beam, will violate the tissue tolerance and results in high complication rates [17]. Methods, including the use of radiosensitizers [18, 19], and hyperthermia [20], to enhance the effect of radiotherapy without increasing the total doses, are presently under evaluation.

Radical surgery consists of two steps: the removal of the uterus, parametria and part of the vagina, and the pelvic lymphadenectomy. These two steps are separate parts of the operation and can also be performed separately. Surgical techniques have been developed which enable us to remove the central organs with a sufficient degree of radicality with acceptable risks. There are, however, definite limitations. The borderline between technically operable and inoperable cases is disputable, but with increasing tumor volume, the radicality needed to clear the central part of the pelvis of the cancerous process, increases the risk of complications to a point where it becomes prohibitive. The Wertheim-type of hysterectomy is sufficiently radical for stages IB and IIA. If the parametria are involved, radicality can no longer be ensured with this technique, and there is general agreement that such patients are best served by treatment with radiotherapy. More radical techniques, like exenterations have been developed, but have no place in the primary treatment of early disease.

Lymph node metastases in stage IA

The rationale for dividing stage I into two subgroups simply according to tumor size is that somewhere along the line of progression from CIN to the generally disseminated disease, it should be possible to delineate a lesion not yet so intimately in contact with the surrounding tissues that vascular

spaces are invaded and viable tumor cells disseminated to other organs. The size of this hypothetical, truly localized lesion is not known.

Reports of treatment results in stage IA are numerous and often given 5-year survival figures as high as 99–100% [21, 22]. The paucity of published materials, uniformly treated and defined, makes it virtually impossible to decide the frequency of lymph node mestastases in this stage of disease. In an extensive survey Benson [23] in 1977, concluded that after excluding biased series, the world literature contained no more than 98 published cases with tumors infiltrating up to 5 mm into the cervical stroma, which had been treated with lymphadenectomy. In this collected series, only one patient had pelvic lymph node metastasis. In a later, presumably unbiased series, Hasumi [24] reported 135 patients with a maximum infiltration depth of 5 mm, all operated with pelvic lymphadenectomy, and he found pelvic spread in five (3.7%). Thus, if stage IA is defined as a tumor with infiltration depth of less than 5 mm, a very modest metastasis rate, presumably less than 5% can be anticipated. The important question is whether all patients who have tumors which conform to this definition should have their pelvic lymph nodes removed or otherwise treated. Radical surgery has a definite mortality risk, but not as high as 5%. Survival, however, is negatively influenced by the presence of lymph node metastases, even when they are removed. Therefore the anticipated improval in survival after surgical removal of metastases, will never equal the metastatic rate found.

Long-term follow-up of patients treated with only local excision of tumor (conization or conservative hysterectomy), represents another approach to the question of optimal treatment for these very early cases. Two such studies have been published, one by Christophersen [25], who found no cancer deaths among 54 patients followed for 10 years after conization or hysterectomy, and one from the Radium Hospital [12]. The estimated 25-year survival of our 108 patients was 97%. Metastases in the pelvic lymph nodes, documented as an isolated pelvic wall recurrence, was encountered in only three patients. Analysis taking the depth of infiltration into account showed that only 1/80 patients (1.3%) with infiltration depths from 1 to 3 mm recurred in contrast to 7.8% when the depth of infiltration was more than 3 mm.

In conclusion the depth of infiltration seems to be a very reliable single prognostic factor suited to make decisions regarding the radicality of the therapeutic procedure. In the absence of lymphatic vessel infiltration, patients with tumors of less than 3 mm infiltration can be treated with a conservative method with à minimal risk of recurrence. Whether this procedure is local eradication (conization or isotope implants) or a simple hysterectomy, will depend on factors such as age, clinical operability, or the preference of the patient for a specific procedure.

Lymph node metastases in stages IB and IIA

The reported incidence of pelvic lymph node metastases in stage IB varies from less than 10% to well over 30% [26, 27]. The prevalence of positive nodes in surgically removed specimens is mainly dependent on two factors; the histological technique and the completeness of the lymphadenectomy.

Obviously the incidence will also vary with the definition and treatment of stage IA. In a series of papers we have shown that between 20 and 25% of all patients in stage IB have pelvic lymph node metastases. In addition approximately 1% has demonstrable spread outside the true pelvis to the para-aortic area. This relatively high incidence of pelvic lymph node involvement is probably linked to our active attitude towards conization thus leaving fewer patients, but with a higher risk of lymphatic spread, in the group treated by radical surgery. In stage IIA only a selected fraction of the patients is operable, and consequently the 'true' incidence of lymphatic dissemination in this stage is unknown. In a series of 62 patients with small IIA tumors [28], metastases were found in 20 (32%). Thus we are able to conclude that in patients who are candidates for radical surgery, dissemination within the treatment area can be expected in well over 25% if routine histological procedures are used. Consequently a very substantial proportion of our patients belong to a potential high risk category.

The prognostic impact of lymph node metastases and the relation of survival to the site of metastases has been studied by Martimbeau [29] who analysed treatment results in 562 patients with squamous cell cancer from the Radium Hospital. He found that patients with spread above the external iliac level had a 5-year survival of only 14% despite maximum treatment including postoperative irradiation. For patients with metastases below the common iliac level no significant difference in survival could be found between the different nodal groups. Nor did it seem to matter whether metastases were found in only one group of nodes or several, or if spread was unilateral or bilateral. The findings of this paper are summarized in

Table 5. Site and frequency of recurrence for 126 patients with pelvic lymph node metastases; stage I B.

			Site of recurrences		
Site of metastases	No.	% of total	Pelvic	Distant	Unknown
Primary nodes	88	70	17 (19%)	12 (14%)	7 (8%)
Secondary nodes	38	30	20 (52%)	7 (18%)	5 (13%)
Total	126		37 (30%)	19 (15%)	12 (10%)

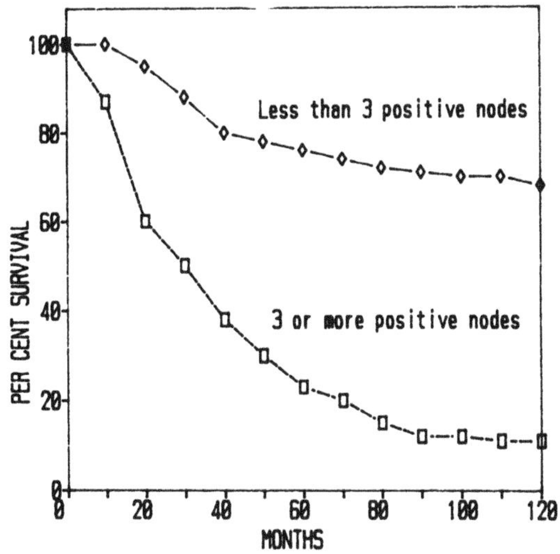

Figure 2. Survival of patients with pelvic lymph node metastases; stage IB.

Table 5. These results can only be interpreted as an evidence of the very serious prognostic significance of any detectable dissemination. A recent study [30] has been directed towards a more detailed study of the prognosis of patients with pelvic lymph node involvement. A multivariate analysis in 300 patients followed for 10 years after operation for stage IB disease showed that the number of metastases found was the most important prognostic criterion. If three or more metastatic nodes were found in the pelvis, the 10-year survival was a modest 12% compared to a 75% survival when the number was less than three. No patient with four or more metastases survived for more than 5 years (Figure 2).

Occult dissemination

Another significant observation from Martimbeau's series was that extrapelvic recurrences were found in 4% of the patients without and in 15% of those with pelvic lymph node metastases. Thus extrapelvic spread at the time of diagnosis can be anticipated in approximately 5–10% of all patients in stage IB.

Diagnosis of the high risk patient

Diagnostic methods include the use of radiology, tumor markers and surgery.

Lymphography

From our institution Kolbenstvedt [31] has published a series of 300 consecutive patients in stages IB and IIA. Pedal lymphography was done in patients who underwent combined treatment with preoperative radium insertions followed 6 weeks later by radical hysterectomy with lymph node dissection. The initial examination was done in conjunction with the intracavitary treatment. Additional X-rays were taken immediately prior to, and also during the operation. The intraoperative radiogram was used to ensure a complete dissection. An X-ray was taken of the removed lymph nodes and, if a lymphographic abnormality was found in the specimen, extra histologic sections were taken from this node. All other nodes were examined by routine procedures. It is appropriate to sum up Kolbenstvedt's findings as the investigation is the most extensive of its kind that has been published:

1. The overwhelming majority (98.9%) of the removed nodes contained contrast medium.
2. All solitary metastases found, were located in regions ordinarily demonstrated by pedal lymphography.
3. Metastases in the parametria were extremely rare, and only seen in two patients.
4. Of a total of 209 lymph nodes, in which metastases were found, 32 (15%) did not contain enough contrast medium to be radiologically detectable.
5. By the aid of the intraoperative lymphogram the surgeon was able to remove an additional 770 lymph nodes (8% of the total yield), which would not have been found otherwise. In these additionally removed glands, metastases were found in 2.7%.

The fact that 15% of all metastatic lymph nodes removed from the pelvis contain too small amounts of contrast medium to be radiologically detectable, shows that this method cannot be trusted in the detection of patients with pelvic lymph node metastases. False positive findings are also common if the criteria for the interpretation of the lymphograms are slack. Contrast medium defects will have to be of a certain size in order to be of significant importance. In a prospective series the reliability of the method has been investigated [32] and very strict criteria for the lymphographic findings was defined. Also in this series, a combined treatment approach was used with a 6-week interval between the intracavitary radiation and the operation. The following criteria were found to be of predictive value:

1. Appearance or growth of a lymph node contrast filling defect during the 6-week period between first and second evaluation; the latter being performed immediately prior to the operation.
2. Nodal defects larger than 10 mm with a sharp outline combined with

signs of altered lymph flow, or surrounded by a distinct rim of contrast medium accumulation ('halo phenomenon').
3. Interruption of lymph flow combined with abnormal collateral lymph vessels.

The results of this investigation are shown in Table 6.

Lymphography is potentially dangerous to patients with allergy towards the contrast medium which is accumulated in the lymphatic system for a long time. This may result in prolonged allergic reactions which are very difficult to cope with.

Because of the large number of false negative findings, lymphography cannot be used as a method to identify patients of the low risk category. Only by repeated examination will it reveal a sufficient number of high risk patients, but in this situation, the specificity is excellent and the method can be helpful in the search for some high risk patients.

Tumor markers

Except for the beta sub unit of CG used in trophoblastic disease, and alpha fetoprotein found in endodermal sinus tumors, we know of no specific markers for patients with gynecologic cancers. This field is rapidly expanding and promising reports in cancer of the ovary [33] have been published. Japanese authors claim to have found a reliable tumor antigen of squamous cell carcinoma, useful in the detection of cervical cancer [34].

Carcinoembryonic antigen (CEA)

During the last decade carcinoembryonic antigen, first described by Gold and Freedman in 1965 [35] has been the most thoroughly studied tumor associated antigen in cervical cancer. It was isolated from, and first believed to be a specific antigen of colonic cancer, but it has later been shown that

Table 6. Lymphographic findings in patients with pelvic lymph node metastases.

	Patients with metastases (%)	
	First evaluation	Second evaluation (after 6 weeks)
Negative	33	30
Uncertain	46	15
Positive	21	55

There were no false positive findings in the second evaluation.

the antigen was common to several different malignancies. Its potential usefulness in cervical cancer was first shown by Khoo and Mackay [36] and later several authors have shown that a relation exists between tumor volume and levels of circulating antigen.

Native CEA from different primary tumors might not be identical and some of the antigenic determinants of the molecule are shared by normal tissue components. This amply demonstrates that the test is not specific. All commerciable available kits employ antibodies derived from colonic cancer and it is possible that CEA extracted from other tumors is sufficiently different to influence the test results. Therefore the antigenic activity found in patients with cervical cancer should perhaps be referred to as 'CEA-like'. Most patients with cervical cancer have plasma values of CEA near the levels found in healthy persons. For this reason the definition of a lower reference value is important for the specificity and sensitivity of the test. Thus if the cut-off level is set too low, the specificity will be low. To compensate for this, a higher cut-off level could be chosen, but the test would then lose much of its sensitivity. Some non-malignant conditions such as inflammatory bowel diseases, as well as pulmonary and liver diseases are associated with increased levels of circulating CEA. Excessive cigarette smoking and old age have also been shown to influence CEA levels. All these factors should be considered when working with the predictive value of CEA, as the incidence of disturbing factors is high in some cancer populations. Patients with cancer of the cervix are relatively young and concomitant diseases are rare. Therefore the number of patients with irrelevant elevation of CEA is low, if a proper cut-off value is chosen.

Specific elevation of CEA is only found in patients with CEA producing tumors. A correlation between tumor content of CEA and the plasma levels has been reported [37], but there is no absolute parallelism. Peripheral plasma values are evidently dependent on other factors that tumor content alone. The metabolism and release mechanisms of this antigen are poorly understood, but important for a full appreciation of the clinical significance of plasma levels.

One of the main problems when working with the clinical relevance of CEA is the reproducibility of the test in the laboratory. The most commonly applied test, the CEA-Roche test of Hansen [38], uses perchloric acid (PCA) extraction followed by dialysis or gel filtration to remove PCA prior to the radioimmunoassay. Performed as recommended the test is sensitive and specific. The extraction and purification procedures are time consuming and delicate and will definitely influence the reproducibility in large scale routine. The PCA extraction is necessary to ensure specificity in the low range and cannot be omitted.

Lack of inter- and intra-assay reproducibility, heterogeneity of studied materials, exaggerated expectations as well as a poor understanding of the influence of concomitant conditions are factors which have discredited the use of CEA determinations, a potentially very powerful test in the detection of subclinical disease.

Diagnostic significance of CEA

Pretreatment values of CEA correspond reasonably well with tumor volume [39]. Therefore it should be theoretically possible to discover subclinical dissemination prior to treatment by the use of this method, and consequently make decisions regarding optimal treatment of a segment of high risk patients. In order to make such decisions it is necessary to define a cut off level which is suitable for the purpose. Different histologic types of tumors have different potential for CEA production or release. In practical use we have found that the predictive significance of pre-treatment values differs for squamous cell carcinomas and adenocarcinomas [40–42]. Adenocarcinomas of the cervix are very reliable CEA producers/releasers and a low pre treatment value practically rules out that the tumor is disseminated beyond the cervix, whereas a low pre-treatment value in squamous cell carcinomas is equivocal. A low value as defined by Hansen *et al.* corresponds to 2.5 μg/l or less. We have found that such a low cut-off level is quite unsuitable in cervical cancer populations because the majority of the patients with early disease will have values near or under the lower limit. The specificity of the test will therefore be uninteresting.

The reliability of the method can be established in operated patients in whom all pelvic lymph nodes were removed for histologic examination. Our experience is summarized in Tables 7 and 8. The cut-off level in these cases was set at 5.0 μg/l. This high cut-off level guarantees a high specificity of the method, but the sensitivity will be low. Until more specific markers are found, this is a necessary compromise. In squamous cell carcinomas approximately 50% of patients with pelvic lymph node metastases had values above this level. In adenocarcinomas seven out of eight patients with pelvic lymph node metastases had elevated levels.

Table 7. CEA in relation to pelvic lymph node metastases in 103 patients with squamous cell carcinoma; stage I B.

	Pretreatment value of CEA in μg/l	
	< 5.0	> 5.0
Total no. of patients	88	15
No. of patients with pelvic lyph node metastases	19 (22%)	9 (60%)

Table 8. CEA in relation to pelvic lymph node metastases in 32 patients with adenocarcinoma of the cervix; stage IB.

	Pretreatment values in µg/l	
	<5.0	>5.0
Total no. of patients	23	9
Patients with pelvic lymph node metastases	1 (4%)	7 (78%)

Prognostic significance of CEA determinations

Dissemination occasionally occurs outside the pelvis without pelvic lymph node involvement. In such cases an elevated CEA level would appear to be false positive at the time of operation. Therefore an estimation of the reliability of the method includes long-term follow-up. We have found that the prognostic significance of elevated pre-treatment levels is very high. Patients with squamous cell cancers in stage IB with pre-treatment levels over 5.0 µg/l have a prognosis similar to patients in stage III, with a recurrence rate of more than 50% at 3 years and an estimated 5-year survival of only 35% (Figure 3). For patients with operable adenocarcinomas in stages IB and IIA, the estimated 5-year survival of patients with CEA levels over 5.0 µg/l is 11%, compared with 90% if values were under this level.

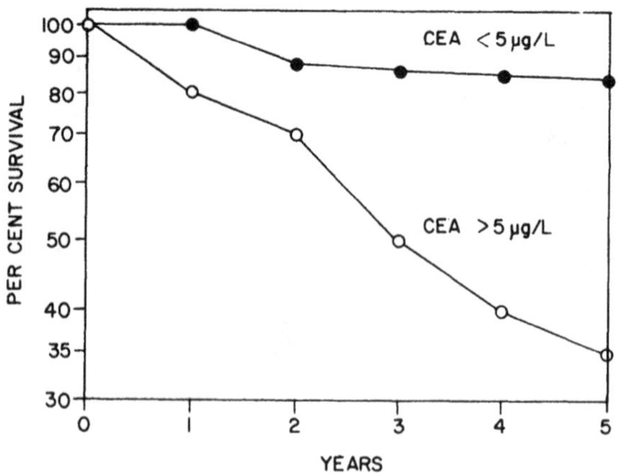

Figure 3. Prognosis of patients with squamous cell carcinoma of the cervix in relation to pre-treatment levels of carcinoembryonic antigen.

Surgery

The depth of infiltration of a tumor is virtually impossible to determine unless the whole tumor is available for examination. In very small tumors a wedge biopsy may be sufficient, but in the majority of cases, a cone specimen is preferred. In order to delineate lesions which do not warrant radical treatment, our therapeutic approach includes a diagnostic cone for any ectocervical tumor which is less than 10 mm in diameter. If care is taken to avoid conizations in patients with endocervical engagement, at least 50% of these small tumors have an infiltration depth of less than 3 mm and further therapy is not necessary if vascular involvement is absent. Tumors with an infiltration depth of more than 3 mm or with vascular involvement are regarded as potential high risk and these patients should be further evaluated for radical treatment with external beam or surgery. Our pathologists are reluctant to diagnose vascular involvement on frozen sections, and a radical procedure immediately following conization is usually not possible. This is of little disadvantage to the patient as the cone is performed by means of a laser beam as an out patient procedure. Laser conizations can be done under sedation or possibly in light anaesthesia and the specimen is ready for examination the next day. Consequently radical treatment, if indicated, can be instituted within 24 or 48 h.

Lymphadenectomy

The finding of metastatic lymph nodes in the pelvis is the most reliable prognostic parameter we know. A complete lymphadenectomy is therefore an important diagnostic procedure in early stages. If postoperative radiotherapy is not used in patients with such metastases, lymphadenectomy also becomes a therapeutic procedure of utmost importance. Cancerous lymph nodes left behind in the pelvis will lead to the development of lateral pelvic wall recurrences and possibly further metastases. These recurrences are extremely difficult to treat and such patients are almost invariably lost.

The use of intraoperative radiograms in patients subjected to lymphography can be very useful in the search for possible lymph nodes left behind after the initial surgical procedure. In the earlier mentioned series by Kolbenstvedt, 8% more lymph nodes were found and removed as a direct consequence of this technique. An absolute complete lymphadenectomy is difficult to accomplish, and could only be achieved in approximately 30% of our patients, despite a maximum effort [43]. The number of lymph nodes left behind in the pelvis, however, had little effect on the long-term prognosis, as long as the number did not exceed three. For patients with 0–3 remaining nodes the 10-year survival was 87% compared with 74% for patients with four or more nodes left in the pelvis after surgery.

The inadequacy of pelvic lymphadenectomy can be estimated from the results in the 80 cases in whom a complete operation was performed. In 6% of these patients pelvic wall recurrences were found and 7.5% relapsed outside the pelvis. These percentages are the same as found in the total material of 300 patients.

Therapeutic consequences

By means of the methods outlined in this chapter, a proportion of high risk patients with early stage disease, can be recognized, either before treatment, or as a part of the treatment procedures. This has a triple purpose. Firstly, patients with low risk can be recognized and offered treatment which is less radical and consequently less risky. This will lead to a lower complication rate but with the same over-all results. Secondly, high risk patients can be given a treatment which is more adequately adapted to their needs and thirdly, subsets of patients with a dismal prognosis can be recogrized in which conventional treatment is clearly ineffective and should be substituted by new treatment concepts. Surgery and radiotherapy are well established methods with only a limited potential for further improvement. Consequently, effective chemotherapy and better diagnostic procedures are urgently needed. Ultimately our work with high risk patients will undoubtedly be of benefit to all patients with cancer of the cervix. Specific tumor markers will probably be detected in a near future and give us a means for monitoring and possibly treating disease, way beyond our present possibilities. These are future aspects, but in the meantime we should concentrate on using our present knowledge to enhance treatment results and minimize damage to our patients.

The important points made in this discussion are summarized in the following general conclusion.

1. The concept of a localized lesion with a minimal potential for dissemination should be accepted and this lesion should be actively searched for. Limited infiltration depth has a prognostic significance of its own, all patients with a macroscopically small tumor should be given the advantage of a diagnostic conization in order to determine if further treatment is indicated. In the absence of lymphatic vessel infiltration, a local procedure is sufficient if the depth of infiltration is less than 3 mm. Increased use of cytology leads to earlier diagnosis and a better stage distribution. Therapists should take maximum advantage of this situation.
2. Patients with tumors with a substantial risk of dissemination should be subjected to diagnostic procedures in order to detect pelvic or distant metastases. If pelvic lymphadenectomy is performed as part of the pri-

mary treatment, it is mandatory that the lymph node dissection is done as complete as possible. Massive involvement of pelvic or para-aortic lymph nodes can be diagnosed and represent a stage of disease which cannot be coped with by means of surgery with or without the addition of external radiotherapy. Any patient with more than three positive pelvic lymph nodes must therefore be considered for alternative treatment. If extra-pelvic spread is suspected because of high pretreatment values of CEA, we should have the courage to treat this suspected dissemination with additional chemotherapy.

3. The excellent results achieved in patients with limited pelvic spread, by means of a combination of radical surgery and postoperative irradiation, clearly indicate that this combination is effective and should be adhered to.
4. Adenocarcinomas of early stages are less curable by radiotherapy alone, and surgery should therefore be considered in all such cases.

References

1. Truelsen F. 1949. Cancer of the uterine cervix. Clinical features with particular reference to the results of radiotherapy. Rosenkilde & Bagger, Copenhagen.
2. Lindell A. 1962. Carcinoma of the uterine cervix. Incidence and influence of age. Acta Radiol (Suppl) 92.
3. Kottmeier HL. 1964. Surgical and radiation treatment of carcinoma of the uterine cervix. Acta Obstet Gynecol Scand (Suppl) 43.
4. Gynning I, Johnsson JE, Alm P, Trope C. 1983. Age and prognosis in Stage IB squamous cell carcinoma of the uterine cervix. Gynecol Oncol 15:18.
5. Kjorstad KE. 1977. Carcinoma of the cervix in the young patient. Obstet Gynecol 50:28.
6. Kjorstad KE. 1977. Adenocarcinoma of the uterine cervix. Gynecol Oncol 5:219.
7. Kjorstad KE, Bond B. 1984. Adenocarcinoma of the cervix, stage IB. Metastatic potential and patterns of dissemination. Am J Obstet Gynecol 150:297.
8. Beecham JB, Halvorsen T, Kolbenstvedt A. 1978. Histologic classification, lymph node metastases and patient survival in Stage IB cervical carcinoma. Gynecol Oncol 6:93.
9. Stendahl U, Willen H, Willen R. 1979. Classification and grading of invasive squamous cell carcinoma of the uterine cervix. Acta Radiol Oncol 18:481.
10. Roche WD, Norris HJ. 1975. Microinvasive carcinoma of the cervix. Cancer 36:180.
11. Larsson G, Alm PO, Gullberg B, Grundsell H. 1983. Prognostic factors in early invasive carcinoma of the uterine cervix. Am J Obstet Gynecol 146:145.
12. Iversen T, Abeler V, Kjorstad KE. 1979. Factors influencing the treatment of patients with stage IA cancer of the cervix. Br J Obstet Gynaecol 85:593.
13. Kjorstad KE. 1984. Early stage cervical cancer. Diagnosis and treatment of high risk patients with particular reference to the use of carcinoembryonic antigen. Thesis, Oslo.
14. Henriksen E. 1949. The lymphatic spread of carcinoma of the cervix and of the body of the uterus. Am J Obstet Gynecol 58:924.
15. Morrow CP. 1980. Is pelvic radiation beneficial in the postoperative management of Stage IB carcinoma of the cervix with pelvic node metastasis treated by radical hysterectomy and pelvic lymphadenectomy? Gynecol Oncol 10:105.

16. Iversen T, Kjorstad KE, Martimbeau PW. 1982. Treatment results in carcinoma of the cervix stage IB in a total population. Gynecol Oncol 14:1.
17. Kjorstad KE, Martimbeau P, Iversen T. 1983. Stage IB carcinoma of the cervix. Urinary and gastrointestinal complications. Gynecol Oncol 15:42.
18. Kjorstad KE, Davy M, Vergote I. Misonidazole in the treatment of advanced squamous cell cervical cancer (in press).
19. Dische S. 1984. MRC trial of misonidazole in carcinoma of the uterine cervix. Br J Radiol 57:491.
20. Surwit E, Manning M *et al.* 1983. Interstitial thermoradiotherapy in recurrent gynecologic malignancies. Gynecol Oncol 15:95.
21. Kolstad P. 1969. Carcinoma of the cervix, Stage IA. Am J Obstet Gynecol 104:1015.
22. Benson WL, Norris HJ. 1977. A critical review of the frequency of lymph node metastasis and death from microinvasive carcinoma. Obstet Gynecol 49:632.
23. Benson WL, Norris HJ. 1977. A critical review of the frequency of lymph node metastasis and death from microinvasive carcinoma. Obstet Gynecol 49:632.
24. Hasumi K, Sakamoto A, Sugano H. 1980. Microinvasive carcinoma of the uterine cervix. Cancer 45:928.
25. Christopherson WM, Gray LA, Parker JE. 1976. Microinvasive carcinoma of the uterine cervix. Cancer 38:629.
26. Rampone JF, Klem V, Kolstad p. 1973. Combined treatment of Stage IB carcinoma of the cervix. Obstet Gynecol 41:163.
27. Fuller AF, Elliot N, Kosloff MS, Lewis JL. 1982. Lymph node metastazses from carcinoma of the cervix, Stages IB and IIA: Implications for prognosis and treatment. Gynecol Oncol 13:165.
28. Kjorstad KE. Combined treatment versus pure radiotherapy in stage IIA cancer of the cervix (in press).
29. Martimbeau P, Kjorstad KE, Iversen T. 1982. Stage IB carcinoma of the cervix. Results when pelvic nodes are involved. Obstet Gynecol 60:215.
30. Kjorstad KE, Kolbenstvedt A. Pelvic lymphadenectomy; a diagnostic or therapeutic procedure? (in press).
31. Kolbenstvedt A. 1975. A lymphographic study of patients with carcinoma of the cervix Stages I and II. Thesis, Universitetsforlaget, Oslo.
32. Kjorstad KE, Drevvatne T, Kolbenstvedt A. 1980. Lymphography and CEA in the diagnosis of metastases in stage IB cancer of the Cervix. Diagn Obstet Gynecol 2:71.
33. Bast R, Klug T, Schaetzl E *et al.* 1984. Monitoring ovarian CA with a combination of CA 125, CA 19-9 and CEA. Am J Obstet Gynecol 149:553–559.
34. Kato H, Morioka H, Tsutsui H. 1982. Value of tumor antigen (TA-4) of squamous cell carcinoma in predicting the extent of cervical cancer. Cancer 50:1294.
35. Gold P, Freedman SO. 1965. Specific carcinoembryonic antigens of the human digestive system. J Exp Med 122:467.
36. Khoo SK, Mackay EV. 1973. Carcinoembryonic antigen in cancer of the female reproductive system: Sequential levels and effect of treatment. Aust N Z Obstet Gynecol 3:1.
37. van Nagell JR, Donaldson ES, Gay EC *et al.* 1979. Carcinoembryonic antigen in carcinoma of the uterine cervix: Tissue localization and correlation with plasma antigen concentration. Cancer 44:944.
38. Hansen HJ, Snyder JJ, Miller E *et al.* 1974. Carcinoembryonic antigen (CEA) assay. A laboratory adjunct in the diagnosis and management of cancer. Human Pathol 5:139.
39. Kjorstad KE, Ørjasaeter H. 1978. CEA levels in patients with squamous cell cancer of the cervix. Obstet Gynecol 51:536.
40. Kjorstad KE, Orjasaeter H. 1982. Prognostic value of CEA determination in plasma of patients with squamous cell cancer of the cervix. Cancer 50:238.

41. Kjorstad KE, Ørjasaeter H. 1984. The prognostic significance of CEA determinations in patients with adenocarcinoma of the cervix. Gynecol Oncol 19:284–289.
42. Kjorstad KE, Ørjasaeter H. 1978. Studies on CEA levels in patients with adenocarcinoma of the uterus. Cancer 40:2953.
43. Kjorstad KE, Kolbentvedt A, Strickert T. 1984. Value of a complete lymphadenectomy in the radical treatment of cancer of the cervix. Cancer 54:2215–2219.

3. Cytosolic estrogen and progesterone receptors in primary cervical carcinoma

LEO B. TWIGGS, ROGER A. POTISH and
BENJAMIN S. LEUNG

Introduction

Steroid hormone action in specific target cells has been under intense study for the last three decades. Refinements in the technique of radioreceptor assay combined with the availability of radio-labeled steroid analogues have increased the precision and sensitivity in the measurement of hormone receptors. These assays were first used as clinical adjuvants in breast and prostate malignancies which are thought of as hormone 'responsive'. In parallel with studies of breast carcinoma, quantification of cytosolic estrogen receptors (ERc) and cytosolic progesterone receptors (PRc) in endometrial carcinoma has been touted as an prognostic index [1–5]. In addition, association of receptor quantity with response to hormone treatment in endometrial carcinoma has been documented [1, 6].

Although cervical carcinoma is not generally considered a hormonally 'responsive' cancer, normal cervical tissue binds radio-labeled estrogen and progesterone, and thus has hormone receptors [7]. Furthermore, the presence of ERc and PRc has also been documented in primary and metastatic cervical cancer tissues [8–10].

The difficulty experienced in assessing the clinical utility of receptor quantity in a number of human cancers may be relative to the goals of the individual investigator. For example, while the basic scientist has as his ideal the unraveling of intracellular mechanisms using receptor measurement as a tool to investigate macromolecular interaction, the clinical scientist evaluates this quantity as a prognostic parameter. Thus, the biochemical classification of neoplastic tissue specifically with ERc and PRc is similar to the more traditional histopathologic and morphologic classifications which are useful in predicting survival and selecting treatment. The central question to the clinical scientist is, 'Can these assays, namely, ERc and PRc, be used to stratify patients treated with the standard regimen to identify those individuals at risk for failure?'. If they can be used in this fashion then

E.A. Surwit, D.S. Alberts (eds) Cervix Cancer.
 ISBN 0-89838-822-8. Printed in the Netherlands.

those patients at high risk for failure may be offered alternative treatment plans and modalities. Our investigations have explored this question by correlating ERc and PRc to traditional prognostic parameters.

Methods and materials

Patients undergoing definitive therapy in the Division of Gynecologic Oncology at the University of Minnesota had cancer tissue excised directly from the primary lesions prior to the onset of therapy. Only cancers which were visible to the naked eye were assayed. A representative section was taken for histopathology to assure that neoplastic tissue was indeed being assayed.

Following excision, tumor specimens were transported to the laboratory immediately and quickly frozen and stored in liquid nitrogen until processed. The methods for homogenization in the presence of 20 mM of sodium molybdate, the preparation of cytosol, and the single saturation point assay by Dextran coated charcoal for ERc and PRc have been described in detail [11, 12]. Tritiated steroids, (2, 4, 6, 7^3, H) 17 B estradiol, 135 ci/mmol for ERc and (6, 7^3, H) progesterone (4 pregnene 3, 20 dione; 55.7 ci/mmol) for PRc were used as ligands and 100 folds excess of diethyl stilbestrol and progesterone were used as competitors, respectively. Protein content of the cytosol was determined by the method of Lowry and associates [13]. Each assay was completed in duplicate or triplicate depending on the amount of tissue available. The intraassay and interassay coefficient of variation were 6 and 8% respectively. The technique is sensitive to 2 fmol/mg cytosolic protein. Correlation of this assay (single saturation point) to the multiple concentration according to Scatchard analysis and sucrose density gradient centrifugation assay were done ($r = 0.85$, $r = 0.86$, respectively). All data included in this report are from the single saturation point method.

Clinical correlates

Mean receptor levels were grouped according to traditional clinical parameters of stage, histologic type and grade, and menopausal status (Table 1). While a slight decrease in mean PRc was seen with increasing clinical stage, small numbers precluded definite conclusions. Little, if any, differences were noted in ERc with respect to clinical stage. Mean levels for both ERc and PRc were relatively consistent within histologic types. Within histologic grade, decreasing PRc levels were noted with dedifferentiation. This trend was less pronounced with ERc. Premenopausal patients relative to postmenopausal patients had a higher mean level of PRc, but not ERc. This is

Table 1. ERc and PRc mean value grouped according to stage, histologic type, grade, and menstrual status.

	PRc (fmol/mg protein)		ERc (fmol/mg protein)	
	Number	Mean	Number	Mean
Total	65	14	61	14
Clinical stage				
I B	44	48	40	14
II A, B	16	31	16	16
III B	5	3	5	9
Histologic type				
Adenocarcinoma	14	60	13	10
Adenosquamous	15	28	13	9
Squamous cell	35	39	34	18
Undifferentiated	1	7	1	6
Histologic grade*				
I	10	80	10	20
II	14	75	13	13
III	30	39	29	15
IV	10	17	8	10
Menstrual				
Premenopausal	50	54	46	14
Postmenopausal	15	23	15	14

* One not graded.

consistent with the known phenomenon of estrogen induction of PRc levels in both *in vivo* and *in vitro* [12, 14].

The use of ERc and PRc as predictors in survival is made convenient by assigning a particular value as either positive or negative. Remembering our original question – can ERc and PRc be used to stratify patients and predict survival following conventional treatment? – assessment of a particular cut-off for positive or negative may be empiric. Using scattergrams of data comparing the level of receptor to survival in two published studies, ERc of 6 fmoles/mg cytosolic protein and PRc of 10 fmoles/mg. of cytosolic protein were defined as discrimination points [10, 15].

As shown in Table 2, 50 to 61% of stage IB, IIA, and IIB carcinomas have positive ERc or PRc. However, although the numbers were small, only 40% of stage IIB carcinomas were ERc positive, and no stage IIIB carcinomas were PRc positive.

Histologic category was compared to receptor status (Table 3). Surprisingly, in the adenocarcinoma group, a larger percentage of adenocarcinomas

Table 2. PRc and ERc in primary cervical carcinoma in relation to clinical stage.

Stage	PRc + (%)	ERc + (%)
I B	61	50
II A, B	56	50
III B	0	40
Total	55	49

Table 3. PRc and ERc in primary cervical carcinoma in relation to histologic type.

Histologic type	PRc + (%)	ERc + (%)
Pure adenocarcinoma	71	23
Squamous differentiation *	52	57

* Squamous cell and adenosquamous.

Table 4. PRc and ERc in primary cervical carcinoma in relation to histologic grade.

Grade Broder's	PRc + (%)	ERc + (%)
I	70	40
II	69	67
III	47	48
IV	60	25

were ERc negative, 77% (10 of 13) than were PRc negative, 29% (4 of 14). In lesions containing squamous differentiation, no difference between percentage of ERc and PRc positivity was apparent (Table 3). Similar findings were seen in a preliminary study [10]. Mean levels of ERc and PRc are generally noted to be greater in cells with glandular differentiation. The fact that more ERc negative tumors are seen in adenocarcinoma probably reflects the empiric discrimination point and may not have any intrinsic biochemical meaning reflecting the use of these assays as clinical predictors of survival.

Receptor status was compared to histologic grade using Broders' criteria (Table 4). Again, in Grade I carcinomas, more were ER negative (60%) than were PRc negative (30%). In the ERc group excluding grade I, a decreased percentage of ERc positive cancers were seen with dedifferentiation. However, no such finding was observed for PRc.

To assess whether ERc and PRc status behaved as independent variables with respect to other parameters, Pearson correlation coefficients were cal-

Table 5. Pearson correlation coefficients: relationship of stage, histology, grade, and menstrual status with PRc and ERc.

Parameter	Stage	Histology	Grade	Menstrual status
PRc + vs. PRc −	−0.21	−0.08	−0.09	0.25
ERc + vs. ERc −	−0.04	0.16	−0.10	0.04

culated (Table 5). Little, if any, correlation was noted, supporting the conclusion that ERc and PRc act as independent variables in these patients.

Survival probabilities

Survival of cervical cancer patients in whom ERc and PRc was assayed was computed by the product-limit analysis according to Kaplan-Meier [16]. Statistical significance was defined at the 0.05 level and the generalized Savage (Mantel-Cox) tests were used [16]. From our previous studies, significant differences were noted relative to PRc in a total group of 39 patients ($p < 0.05$) (PRc depicted) (Figure 1) [10]. The difference in survival relative to receptor status was most notable in the premenopausal group ($p < 0.05$) (Figure 2) [10]. No difference in survival relative to receptor status was seen

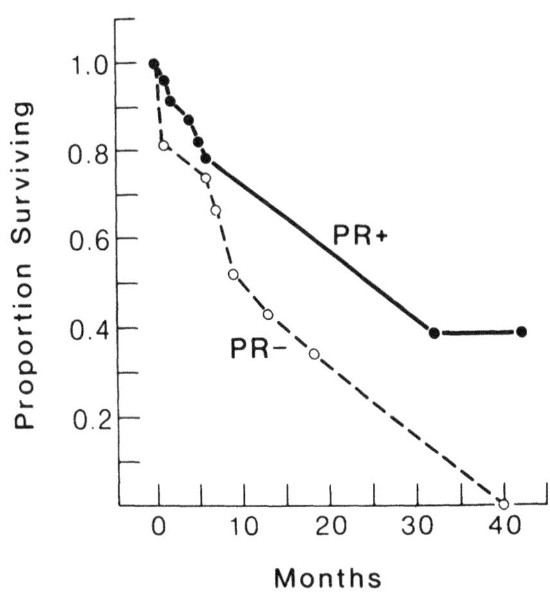

Figure 1. Proportion of primary cervical cancer patients surviving in months grouped according to receptor status in 39 patients. Source: Gao, Twiggs, Leung *et al.* [10].

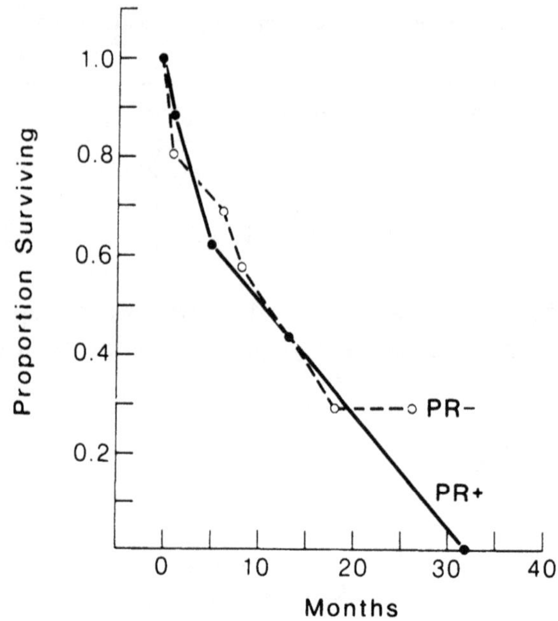

Figure 2. Proportion of postmenopausal cervical cancer patients surviving in months grouped according to progesterone receptor status in 19 patients. Source: Gao, Twiggs, Leung *et al.* [10].

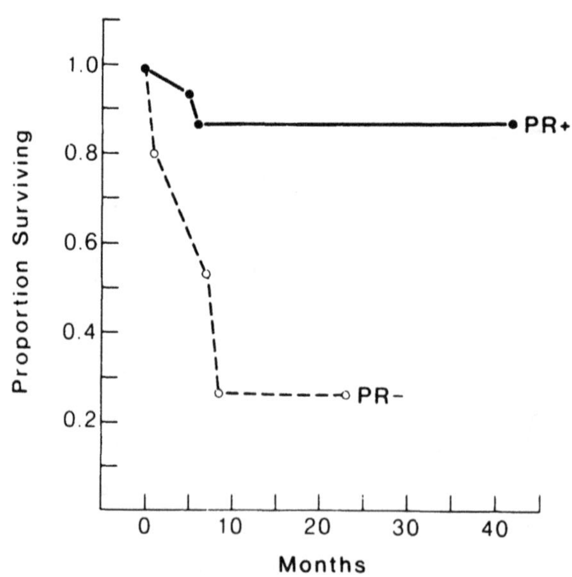

Figure 3. Proportion of premenopausal cervical cancer patients surviving in months grouped according to receptor status in 20 patients. Source: Gao, Twiggs, Leung *et al.* [10].

in the post-menopausal group (Figure 3) [10]. It appears, then, that ERc and PRc are predictors of survival in premenopausal cervical carcinoma patients. The probability in our group of 20 patients with PRc positive cancers of surviving 40 months was 0.9. In contrast, if the PRc assay was negative, the probability of survival at 24 months dropped to 0.3.

These preliminary data were somewhat controversial and have been subject to much discussion. The treatment differences in either group could have skewed the receptor positive group towards better survival or a relatively large group of good prognosis patients could have been present in the receptor positive group. Therefore, another study looking in more detail at homogenously treated stage IB cervical carcinoma noted statistically significant differences in survival relative to receptor status [17]. In this group, ERc status became important and a statistically significant difference in survival relative to ERc was observed [17]. No significant differences were noted relative to receptor status with regards to age, and histologic grade and type. The number of patients with documented nodal metastatic disease prior to treatment were similar in each receptor status group [17].

In a further study, the predictive utility of receptor status along with other prognostic factors was assessed using the proportional hazard regression model of Cox [15]. Again, using this sophisticated statistical maneuver, premenopausal patients with either positive PRc or positive ERc or in combination, had statistically significant differences in survival relative to their receptive negative counterparts. Interestingly, in the total group of patients, no significant differences in survival were noted relative to traditional clinical characteristics such as menopausal status, age, treatment type, histopathologic type and grade, or lymph node involvement. In these ongoing studies, receptor status has prognostic significance and such information is additive to standard clinical and surgical staging procedures [15].

Clinical utility and future directions

Especially, in the premenopausal patient with cervical carcinoma in our patient population receptor status has a prognostic significance and predictive power. As this group of patients had visible cancers, such selection skews the studied groups to poorer prognosis and therefore, assists in the demonstration of the clinical utility of ERc and PRc. To extrapolate these findings to a group of smaller microscopic diagnosed carcinomas may not be warranted. Importantly, while investigations are currently underway in these types of patients, large numbers of patients will be necessary to demonstrate the utility of ERc and PRc for microscopic carcinomas, as survival in these smaller lesions is better.

At present, there are limitations on the utility of these assays. The test, while not extremely expensive, does have a turn around time, which adds to treatment delay. Also, widespread application is not possible as single point saturation assay via the Dextran-coated charcoal method is still methodologically difficult and requires expensive laboratory equipment. Also, fresh frozen tissue is necessary, archiving is not possible and all investigations need be prospective. Furthermore, there remains no reliable standardization for interlaboratory correlation of receptor values. These problems limit these assays' prospective use in treatment planning.

However, the recent development of monoclonal antibodies to the significant portion of the receptor macromolecule combined with immunocytochemical techniques, namely immunoperoxidase staining, may simplify receptor assessments. Although not quantitative, such a technique allows us the luxury of assaying microscopic carcinomas and identifying small clusters of receptor positive cells among large populations of receptor negative cells in some cancers. These factors may result in more widespread usage of receptor quantification. Also, archiving is possible as paraffin stored tissue may be retrospectively studied and correlated to known survival. Currently, studies correlating the monoclonal antibody immunoperoxidase technique with our single point assay are ongoing.

Acknowledgements

National Cancer Institute Research Grant R01-CA259981.

Award to B.S. Leung and the Therese Knutson, Memorial Cancer Fund Fraternal Order of the Eagles Minnesota AERIE # 34; John L. McKelvey, Gynecologic Oncology Registry; Barbara Glubka, Registrar; Susan Greer, for editorial assistance.

References

1. Creasman WT, McCarty KS Sr, Barton TK, McCarty KS Jr. 1980. Clinical correlates of estrogen and progesterone-binding proteins in human endometrial adenocarcinoma. Obstet Gynecol 55:363.
2. Liao BS, Twiggs LB, Leung BS, Potish RA, Prem KA, Yu WY. Cytoplasmic estrogen and progesterone receptors as prognostic parameters in primary endometrial carcinoma. Obstet Gynecol (in press).
3. Horwitz KB, McGuire WL, Pearson OH, Segaloff A. 1975. Predicting response to endocrine therapy in human breast cancer: A Hypothesis. Science 189:726.
4. Degenshein GA, Bloom N, Tobin E. 1980. The value of progesterone receptor assays in the management of advanced breast cancer. Cancer 46:2789.
5. Kiang DT, Frenning DH, Goldman AI, Ascensao VF, Kennedy BJ. 1978. Estrogen receptors and responses to chemotherapy and hormonal therapy in advanced breast cancer. N Engl J Med 299:1330.

6. Ehrlich CF, Young PCM, Cleary RE. 1981. Cytoplasmic progesterone and estradiol receptors in normal, hyperplastic and carcinomatous endometria: Therapeutic implications. Am J Obstet Gynecol 141:539.
7. Sanborn BM, Held B, Kuo HS. 1976. Hormonal action in human cervix. II. Specific progesterone binding proteins in human cervix. J Steroid Biochem 7:665.
8. Terenius L, Lindell A, Persson BH. 1971. Binding of estradiol-17B to human cancer tissue of the female genital tract. Cancer Res 31:1895.
9. Hahnel R, Martin JD, Masters AM, Ratajczak T, Twada.waddle E. 1979. Estrogen receptors and blood hormone levels in cervical carcinoma and other gynecological tumors. Gynecol Oncol 8:226.
10. Gao YL, Twiggs LB, Leung BS, Yu WCY, Potish RA, Okagaki T, Adcock LL, Prem KA. 1983. Cytoplasmic estrogen and progesterone receptors in primary cervical carcinoma: Clinical and histopathologic correlates. Am J Obstet Gynecol 146:299.
11. Leung BS, Fletcher WS, Lindell TS, Wood DC, Krippaehne WW. 1973. Predictability of response to endocrine ablation in advanced breast carcinoma: A correlation to estrogen receptor and steroid sulfurylation, Arch Surg 106:515.
12. Yu WCY, Leung BS, Gao YL. 1981. Effects of estradiol-17B on progesterone receptors and the uptake of thymidine in human breast cancer cell line. CAMA-1, Cancer Res 41:5004.
13. Lowry OH, Rosebrough NJ, Farr AL, Randall RJ. 1981. Protein measurement with the folin phenol reagent. J Biol Chem 193:265.
14. Natrajan PK, Muldoon TG, Greenblatt RB, Mahesh VB. 1982. The effects of progestins on estrogen and progesterone receptors in human endometrium. J Reprod Med 27:227.
15. Potish RA, Twiggs LB, Adcock LL, Prem KA, Savage JE, Leung BS. Prognostic importance of progesterone and estrogen receptors in cancer of the uterine cervix. Cancer (in press).
16. Lee ET. 1980. Statistical Methods for Survival Data Analysis. Lifetime Learning Publications, Belmont, CA.
17. Twiggs LB, Potish RA, Adcock LL, Savage JE, Carson LF, Leung BS. Cytosolic estrogen and progesterone receptors as prognostic parameters in stage IB cervical carcinoma. Gynecol Oncol (in press).

4. Surgical staging of cervical cancer

NEVILLE F. HACKER and JONATHAN S. BEREK

Introduction

Cervical cancer spreads initially by direct extension to the corpus, vagina, and parametrium, and by lymphatic embolization to the pelvic lymph nodes. From the pelvic nodes (external iliac, obturator, and hypogastric) disease disseminates to the common iliac, presacral and paraaortic nodes, and finally via the thoracic duct to the left scalene nodes and the systemic circulation. Rarely, tumors may spread via the posterior cervical trunk directly into the common iliac and paraaortic nodes [1, 2]. Although hematogenous spread occurs, it is usually a relatively late phenomenon in cercical cancer.

In spite of the ready accessibility of the cervix for diagnostic studies, over 50% of patients with cervical cancer have parametrial involvement at the time of diagnosis, making primary surgical therapy inadvisable. Radiation therapy is capable of sterilizing quite bulky primary disease, and has also been shown capable of sterilizing lymph nodes metastases [3, 4]. However, geographic failures will occur with radiation therapy unless all involved lymph nodes are included in the treatment field.

The inability of noninvasive diagnostic studies to detect small lymph node mestastases led many investigators in the 1970s to undertake pretreatment staging laparomoties in order to identify patients with positive paraaortic nodes. These patients were then treated with extended field radiation, to encompass the involved nodes. Over a decade of experience with staging laparotomies for cervix cancer and extended field radiation for patients with positive paraaortic nodes permits a critical evaluation of the current role of this therapeutic approach.

E.A. Surwit, D.S. Alberts (eds) Cervix Cancer.

Non-invasive diagnostic studies

The ideal method for the detection of paraaortic lymph node metastases in genital tract malignancies would be easy to perform, without significant morbidity, and of high sensitivity and specificity, thereby obviating the need for surgical exploration in all patients. Unfortunately, no currently available method meets all of these requirements.

Standard noninvasive studies to detect paraaortic lymph node metastases include the bipedal lymphangiogram, abdominal computed tomography (CT scan), and abdominal ultrasound. More recently, magnetic resonance scanning and monoclonal-antibody imaging have been introduced and may ultimately prove to be more sensitive tests.

Bipedal lymphagiogram

Lymphography gained popularity in the United States in the 1960s. The initial enthusiasm for these studies has subsequently been tempered, as increasing experience has revealed that small metastatic deposits cannot be discerned, and the images demonstrated are frequently nonspecific [5].

The radiologic diagnosis of metastases is based on various criteria which can be classified into two main groups: direct and indirect [6].

Direct signs, which are best observed on 24 to 48 h films include (1) a marginal filling defect in a node, and (2) absence of a node or of a lymphatic group because of total tumor replacement. Indirect signs are mainly noted on the immediate post injection films. They include (1) collateral circulation, (2) displacement of lymphatic channels, (3) blockage of the lymphatic

Table 1. Results of lymphangiography for detection of paraaortic lymph node metastases from cervical cancer.

	Lympangiograms									
Study	No.	Pos.	Neg.	TP	TN	FP	FN	Spec (%)	Sens (%)	Accuracy (%)
Piver (1973) [8]	26	6	20	5	18	1	2	95	71	88.5
Littman (1973) [9]	10	1	9	0	8	1	1	89	0	80.0
Wallace (1977) [7]	89	14	75	14	69	0	6	100	70	93.3
Brown (1979) [10]	21	13	8	5	7	8	1	47	83	57.1
Lagasse (1979) [11]	95	16	79	9	70	7	9	91	50	83.2
Kilcheski (1981) [12]	23	10	13	8	11	2	2	85	70	82.6
Total	264	60	204	41	183	19	21	91	66	84.8

TP = true positive; TN = true negative; FP = false positive; FN = false negative; Spec = specifity; Sens = sentivity.

flow, (4) extravasation, and (5) stasis lasting longer than 24 h. The finding of a filling defect in a lymph node not traversed by lymphatics is the single most reliable criterion for the diagnosis of metastatic carcinoma [7]. False positive readings occur because benign conditions such as fatty degeneration, fibrosis, or periadenitis, may similate a malignant process, and there may also be a congenital absence of a group of nodes. False negative results occur because a metastasis has to be several millimeters in size before it can be recognized with any accuracy.

Results of bipedal lymphangiograms for the evaluation of paraaortic lymph nodes in patients with cervical cancer are shown in Table 1. The overall accuracy of lymphangiograms is about 85%, but the false-positive rate is almost 32% (19 of 60 positive studies), and the false-negative rate about 10% (21 of 204). This implies that reliance should not be placed on lymphangiography alone to determine the need for extended field radiation.

Computed tomography

Computed tomography has been used to help stage pelvic cancers since about 1975. It is a noninvasive test, and a pelvic and abdominal CT scan allows evaluation of not only the lymph nodes but also the primary tumor, liver, urinary tract, and bony structures. Unlike lymphangiograms, which can define alterations in nodal architecture, computed tomography can detect only changes in the size of the nodes. It will identify those enlarged nodes totally replaced by tumor which are not visualized by lymphangiography. Retroperitoneal fat improves the resolution of the paraaortic nodes.

Table 2. Results of CT scans for the detection of paraaortic lymph node metastases from cervical cancer.

Study	CT scans									Accuracy
	No.	Pos.	Neg.	TP	TN	FP	FN	Spec (%)	Sens (%)	(%)
Photopulos (1979) [14]	17	6	11	6	7	0	4	100	60	76.5
Brenner (1982) [15]	20	5	15	4	13	1	2	93	67	85.0
Whitley (1982) [16]	18	5	13	4	12	1	1	92	80	88.9
Villasanta (1983) [17]	42	14	28	10	25	4	3	86	77	83.3
Bandy(1985) [18]	44	12	32	9	29	3	3	91	75	86.4
Total	141	42	99	33	86	9	13	90.5	71.7	84.4

TP = true positive; TN = true negative; FP = false postive; FN = false negative; Spec = specificity; Sens = sensitivity.

Nodes which are enlarged because of inflammatory or hyperplastic changes will give false-positive results. This is a particular problem in cervical cancer, which is frequently associated with secondary infection and enlarged, reactive nodes. Normal-sized nodes containing microscopic tumor deposits will give false-negative results.

Positive findings on CT scan include (1) mattered or multinodular collections of nodes, (2) discrete nodes greater than 1.5 cm in diameter, (3) obliteration by mass of the normal fat planes between the aorta and inferior vena cava [13]. Lymphangiography prior to CT is helpful in definitely establishing an opacified structure to be a lymph node. If nodes smaller than 1.5 cm in diameter are considered positive, the sensitivity of the test will be improved at the expense of the specificity.

Results of computed tomography for the evaluation of paraaortic lymph nodes in patients with cervical cancer are shown in Table 2. They indicate that the sensitivity and specificity of computed tomography for the detection of paraaortic lymph nodes in cervical cancer are comparable to those of lymphangiography. The false-positive rate is approximately 21% (nine of 41 positive readings) and the false-negative rate about 13% (13 of 99). Based on these findings, most authorities recommend that a CT scan be done prior to, or in lieu of lymphangiography, because the test is noninvasive, less time consuming, less technically difficult, and provides more information [12, 18, 19].

Ultrasonography

Ultrasonography is capable of detecting enlarged lymph nodes, particularly those 2 cm or greater in diameter. It is probably of comparable efficacy to computerized tomography, although comparative data are not available for patients with cervical cancer. As with computed tomography, ultrasonography is unable to differentiate between benign and malignant enlargement of lymph nodes but has the advantage of being less costly, less time-consuming, and avoiding any risk from radiation. Either gray-scale B-mode or real-time ultrasound may be used. Difficulty may be experienced in examining the retroperitoneum by ultrasound due to the presence of bowel gas [20].

Monoclonal-antibody imaging

Recently, detection of metastatic carcinoma in normal sized retroperitoneal nodes from a colon primary has been reported using imaging with radiolabeled monoclonal-antibodies [21]. Although not yet reported for cervical cancer, this technology may eventually prove to be the most sensitive non-operative technique for the detection of paraaortic lymph node metastases.

Magnetic resonance imaging

Magnetic resonance imaging (MRI) is also a recent innovation. Its role has not yet been adequately evaluated for gynecologic malignancies. Bies and colleagues reported three patients with paraaortic lymph node metastases from cervical cancer. CT and MRI demonstrated the lymphadenopathy in two of the three, but the third patient, who had microscopic involvement only, was identified only at surgery [22].

Fine needle aspiration cytology of abnormal paraaortic nodes

Percutaneous fine needle aspiration has been widely used for obtaining tissue from many organs, including breast, liver, prostate, and pancreas. The successful aspiration of intraabdominal lymph nodes guided by lymphangiography and fluoroscopy was first reported in 1976 [23]. The fine needle may also be directed by computed tomography or ultrasound. The technique is performed under local anesthesia and is free of major complications, even in the presence of clotting problems. McDonald and colleagues at the University of Michigan reported technically successful fine needle aspirations in 50 of 56 patients (89.3%) with lymphangiographically suspicious pelvic or paraaortic lymph nodes, using fluoroscopic guidance [24]. Not all of their cases with a negative fine needle aspiration were surgically explored, but they estimated the overall diagnostic accuracy of the technique to be 74.0%. Zornosa and colleagues of the M.D. Anderson Hospital reported a diagnostic accuracy of 82% in a series of 72 patients having percutaneous fine needle aspiration of pelvic and paraaortic lymph nodes under fluroroscopic control [25].

Only a positive aspiration should be used as a basis for therapeutic decisions. Patients with a negative aspiration should be subjected to surgical exploration, if appropriate.

Operative staging

Operative staging for cervical cancer is performed in patients in whom the disease is apparently confined to the pelvis after the usual metastatic work-up has been completed. The metastatic work-up should include a chest X-ray, pelvic and abdominal CT scan, skeletal X-rays if there are symptoms of bone pain, cytoscopy, and proctoscopy. Performance of a pelvic and abdominal CT scan obviates the need for an intravenous pyelogram. If the CT scan is negative for metastatic disease, a bipedal lymphangiogram may be performed.

The surgical approach to the retroperitoneal nodes may be either transperitoneal or extraperitoneal, although the latter is associated with less subsequent radiation-induced morbidity.

Transperitoneal approach

The abdomen is opened through a lower midline or paramedian incision, which extends about 3 cm above the umbilicus. After entering the peritoneal cavity, thorough exploration of the abdominal cavity is carried out, pelvic washings taken for cytology, and any suspicious areas biopsied.

The peritoneum is then opened over the bifurcation of the aorta, and extended cephalad for about 5 cm. The small bowel mesentery is retracted, and the aorta and vena cava visualized. Any enlarged nodes are removed and sent for frozen section. If there are no enlarged nodes, or if the frozen section is negative, the fatty tissue containing the lymph nodes anterior and lateral to the vena cava and aorta is dissected en bloc, below the origin of the inferior mesenteric artery. Prior to this dissection, it is important to identify and retract each ureter laterally. The common iliac nodes are also removed, as are any grossly enlarged pelvic nodes below this level.

Extraperitoneal approach

The extraperitoneal approach for the surgical staging of patients with cervical cancer was first described by Berman and colleagues from UCLA in 1977 [26]. Although originally described through a left lateral J-shaped incision, we now use a lower midline incision as described above, which more readily facilitates access to both sides of the pelvis.

Prior to the node dissection, the peritoneum is opened anteriorly and thorough abdominal exploration is carried out as described above. After closing the peritoneum, it is rolled off the anterior abdominal wall to expose the pelvic side wall. The round ligament on each side is ligated and cut to facilitate exposure. As the peritoneum is rolled off the abdominal wall by a combination of sharp and blunt dissection, the inferior epigastric vessels may be followed to allow ready identification of the external iliac artery. On the left side, the retroperitoneum is sufficiently dissected to fully expose the left common iliac vessels. The pararectal and paravesical spaces can be readily developed to allow digital exploration of the parametrium. The left ureter is identified attached to the peritoneum, and is retracted medially. The left common iliac lymph nodes are dissected and submitted. Any enlarged external iliac, hypogastric or obturator nodes on the left side are removed and sent as separate specimens, but full pelvic lymphadenectomy is not performed.

In a similar fashion, the right pelvic side wall is exposed, but the peritoneal retraction is carried further cephalad to expose the inferior vena cava and aorta. As on the left side, the parametrium should be digitally evaluated after development of the pararectal and paravesical spaces, and any enlarged pelvic nodes resected. After medial retraction of the right ureter, any enlarged paraaortic or right common iliac lymph nodes are excised and sent for frozen section. If there are no enlarged nodes, or if the frozen sections are negative, right common iliac and paraaortic nodes are resected en bloc up to the level of origin of the inferior mesenteric artery. Only enlarged nodes above this level need be resected. After this dissection, a Jackson-Pratt drain is placed in the retroperitoneum, brought out through a separate stab incision in the right iliac fossa, and the abdomen closed.

Operative complications

Surgical complications from either approach are infrequent in the hands of an experienced surgeon. The most common serious complication is damage to the great vessels, particularly the inferior vena cava, causing massive hemmorrhage. Delgado reported that four of 86 patients (4.7%) required repair of the inferior vena cava following lymphadenectomy [27]. Ureteric injury is possible if the ureters are not identified prior to the dissection. It is also possible to avulse the inferior mesenteric artery, necessitating its ligation, but because of the anastomoses from the marginal artery, this does not compromise the blood supply to the distal colon unless the patient already has advanced arterial disease. In the Gynecologic Oncology Group (GOG) report of 290 patients, the operative mortality was 0.3% (one case), intraoperative injuries to the vein or ureter occurred in four cases (1.6%) and postoperative urinary fistula or bowel obstruction occurred in seven patients (2.9%) [28].

Incidence of positive paraaortic nodes

Most reports on the incidence of paraaortic lymph nodes in stage I carcinoma of the cervix are biassed by patient selection. However, in the GOG study, all patients with stage I disease had paraaortic lymph node biopsies, and the incidence of positive nodes was 5.6% (eight of 143 cases) [28]. This is similar to the 7% incidence reported from the University of Miami (11 of 155 cases) [29]. For patients with stage II cervical cancer, the incidence of positive paraaortic nodes is about 17% (Table 3), while for patients with stage III disease, the incidence is about 28% (Table 4). In the GOG Study, histologic grade did not significantly influence the incidence of paraaortic nodal metastases, but histologic type seemed to be important [28]. Paraaortic nodal metastases were present in four of 12 patients (33%) with adenocarcinomas, compared with 43 of 258 patients (17%) with squamous carcinomas. This was considered more significant because 75% of the patients with adenocarcinoma had stage 1B disease. However, the number of adenocarcinomas is too small to draw conclusions.

Table 3. Incidence of paraaortic nodal mentastases in stage II cervical cancer.

Study	Explored	Positive	Percent
Nelson (1977) [30]	63	9	14.3
Delgado (1977) [27]	18	8	44.4
Wharton (1977) [31]	57	10	17.5
Piver (1977) [32]	46	6	13.0
Sudarsanam (1978) [29]	43	7	16.3
Buchsbaum (1979) [33]	19	1	5.3
Hughes (1980) [34]	80	14	17.5
Ballon (1981) [35]	48	9	18.8
Welander (1982) [36]	63	13	20.6
Berman (1984) [37]*	265	43	16.2
Potish (1985) [38]	47	5	10.6
Total	749	125	16.7

* Includes GOG patients reported by Lagasse *et al.* [28].

Table 4. Incidence of paraaortic nodal metastases in stage III cervical cancer.

Study	Explored	Positive	Percent
Nelson (1977) [30]	39	15	38.5
Delgado (1977) [27]	13	5	38.5
Piver (1977) [32]	49	18	36.7
Sudarsanam (1978) [29]	19	3	15.8
Buchsbaum (1979) [33]	104	34	32.7
Hughes (1980) [34]	96	23	24.0
Ballon (1981) [35]	24	4	16.7
Welander (1982) [36]	38	10	26.3
Berman (1984) [37]*	180	45	25.0
Potish (1985) [38]	11	4	36.4
Total	573	161	28.1

* Includes GOG patients reported by Lagasse *et al.* [28].

In addition to identifying patients with positive paraaortic lymph nodes, operative staging may identify occult peritoneal spread. In the Memorial Sloan-Kettering Study, 16 of 127 patients (12.6%) undergoing surgical staging had metastatic disease within the peritoneal cavity [36]. Surgical staging may also occasionally demonstrate less tumor than suspected clinically, particularly in patients with undiagnosed endometriosis [26].

Extended field radiation

For patients with positive common iliac or paraaortic lymph nodes, the usual pelvic radiation field is extended to the level of the 12th thoracic vertebra. The width of this extended portal is sufficient to encompass the lateral extent of the transverse processes of the vertebral bodies, and is usually 8 cm in diameter. These patients receive 4500–5000 rad of external radiation to the extended field over 5 weeks, through parallel-opposed antero-posterior and postero-anterior portals.

In a few centers, intraoperative irradiation of involved paraaortic lymph nodes with electron beams has been tried. Limited data are available on this approach and the capability for intraoperative radiation is not available in most centers. There are several advantages to this approach [39]. Firstly, the treatment field can be visualized, so the distribution of the radiation should be more accurate. Secondly, the normal organs, particularly the small bowel, can be shifted out of the treatment beam, thus eliminating radiation-induced small bowel complications. Finally, the use of the electron beam makes it possible to deliver a sufficiently high dose to the lymph nodes without affecting the underlying tissues. The major disadvantage is that the radiation is limited to a single treatment, and the dose must be smaller than the tolerance dose of normal organs which cannot be shifted out of the field. Goldson and colleagues reported using a one-time dose of 2000 rad delivered in 4 min with an electron beam energy source of 6 meV. The only patient reported was free of complications 3 months after treatment.

Complications of radiation therapy following surgical staging

Acute tolerance to extended field radiation is satisfactory. Nausea, vomiting, diarrhea, and weight loss are common during treatment, and may necessitate a brief, temporary interruption of therapy [40]. However, it is rare to have to discontinue treatment because of acute toxicity.

Extended field radiation following surgical staging has been associated with significant long-term morbidity and some mortality. Morbidity has been mainly related to bowel complications such as small bowel obstruction, ileocutaneous fistula, ileovesicle fistula, ileocolic fistula, bowel perforation, radiation enteritis, gastric ulceration and protosigmoiditis.

As increasing experience has accumulated with the use of extended field radiation, it is clear that the single most important factor associated with the increased morbidity is the radiation dose to the extended field [40, 41]. Piver and colleagues reported an intestinal complication rate of 61.9% among 21 patients treated with 6000 rad of split-course radiation in 8 weeks to the paraaortic area, compared to a rate of 10% among ten patients who received 4400 to 5000 rad in 4 1/2 to 5 weeks [42].

A second important factor related to post-radiation morbidity is the type of operative approach. The extraperitoneal approach is associated with significantly less risk of adherent, fixed bowel loops postoperatively, and hence a decreased morbidity. The first 33 patients undergoing surgical staging for cervical cancer at UCLA were operated via a transperitoneal approach and ten of these patients (30.3%) developed small bowel complications requiring surgical correction from 1 to 17 months postoperatively. The complications included enterovaginal fistulas in five patients, small bowel obstruction in nine, and radiation enteritis in six. None of the complications were related to recurrent cancer, but two patients (6%) died as a direct result of the complications [26]. Subsequently, we have performed over 80 staging laparotomies via an extraperitoneal approach, and only one patient has developed a small bowel obstruction, which settled with conservative management.

Wharton and colleagues reported severe postradiation intestinal complications in 32 of 120 operated patients (27%), with death in 16 patients (13%), following a transperitoneal surgical staging [31]. Only 24 of the 120 patients had extended field radiation, to a total dose of 5500 rad. Small bowel obstruction developed in seven patients, three of whom died. Five patients were noted at laparotomy to have loops of small bowel adherent to

Table 5. Survival after extended field radiation.

Study	Patients	5-year survival (%)
Buchsbaum (1979) [33]	21	23.8
Hughes (1980) [34]	22	29.0
Ballon (1981) [35]	18	23.0
Piver (1981) [42]	31	9.6
Welander (1982) [36]	31	25.8
Rubin (1984) [43]*	14	57.1
Potish (1985) [38]	17	40.0
Total	154	26.6

* All had stage I B or II A disease.

the pelvic lymphadenectomy incision areas, with necrosis and perforation of the adjacent segments. Four of the patients dying with intestinal complications were receiving chemotherapy, including adriamycin, for recurrent cancer when the fatal bowel complication occurred.

Prognosis

A number of papers have presented survival data for patients with cervical cancer having extended field radiation for positive paraaortic nodes. These are summarized in Table 5. Most of the data are 5-year survivals, indicating that about one in four patients can be salvaged with this approach.

Sites of recurrence

As shown in Table 6, 39.2% of patients who recur following extended field radiation have distant metastases beyond the radiation field, indicating that for many patients, paraaortic nodal spread heralds systemic disease. Buchsbaum reported that eight of 23 patients (34.8%) with positive paraaortic nodes had positive supraclavicular nodes [33]. Welander and colleagues reported that of 31 patients with positive paraaortic nodes, 17 (54.8%) later developed distant metastases, compared with only 24 of 96 patients (25%) with negative paraaortic nodes ($P < 0.05$) [36]. In the COG experience, 32 of 90 patients (35.5%) with positive paraaortic nodes and a documented site of recurrence developed distant metastases [37].

The second major problem for cervical cancer patients with positive paraaortic nodes is failure to control the pelvic disease. As shown in Table

Table 6. Sites of recurrence in patients with cervical cancer having extended field radiation for positive paraaortic nodes.

Study	Patients	Distant metastases	Percent	Pelvic recurrences	Percent
Nelson (1977) [30]	23	12	52	Not stated	
Piver (1981) [32]	31	14	45	Not stated	
Welander (1982) [36]	31	17	55	12	38
Tewfik (1982) [44]	23	10	44	5	22
Potish (1983) [40]*	81	25	31	16	20
Berman (1984) [37]	90	32	36	25	28
Rubin (1984) [43]	14	5	36	2	14
Total	293	115	39.2	60/239	25.1

* Diagnosis of paraaortic metastases based on lymphangiogram.

6, 25% of patients having extended field radiation for positive paraaortic nodes develop a recurrence in the pelvis.

Current status of surgical staging

Critical review of the experience with surgical staging for cervical cancer indicates that the operation itself is relatively safe, and provided the dose of radiation to the paraaortic field does not exceed 5000 rad, the long-term morbidity following the radiation is not excessive. In fact, if the surgical staging is performed via an extraperitoneal appraoch, the post-radiation morbidity is low.

As a routine procedure, surgical staging has failed to realize its intended goal of substantially improving survival, although it has provided valuable data on the biological behavior of cervical cancer. There are two principle reasons for this unrealized expectation. Firstly, patients with positive paraaortic nodes frequently have occult distant metastases, and as yet, there is no effective adjuvant systemic chemotherapy for cervical cancer. Secondly, failure to control the pelvic disease has contributed significantly to the poor overall survival for this group of patients. In fact, Welander and colleagues at Memorial Sloan-Kettering found no statistically significance difference in survival between patients with negative paraaortic nodes treated with pelvic radiation, and those with positive paraaortic nodes treated with extended field radiation, suggesting that causes of death are related primarily to uncontrolled pelvic disease [36].

In spite of these shortcomings, a 26.6% long-term survival for patients with positive paraaortic nodes is sufficient justification for continued employment of this approach in selected patients, because without the extended field radiation it is unlikely that any of these patients would have survived. Hughes and colleagues reported 17 patients with positive paraaortic nodes who were treated with standard pelvic radiation only, and all were dead by 38 months [34].

Patients likely to derive the most significant survival benefit from surgical staging are those whose primary tumors are small enough for good local control. These patients are, of course, also the ones that will have the lowest incidence of positive nodes, although Hughes and colleagues reported positive paraaortic nodes in five of 19 patiens (26.3%) with stage 1B tumors 6 cm or greater in diameter [34]. Tewfik and colleagues reported prolonged survival in two of five patients (40%) with stage 1B, IIA, or IIB disease, compared to only three of 18 patients (16.6%) with stage IIIB or IVA disease [44]. Rubin and colleagues reported long-term survival in eight of 14 patients (57%) with positive paraaortic nodes and early stage (IB or IIA) disease [43].

Although the data are conflicting [37], the other group of patients likely to derive maximal benefit from surgical staging are those with microscopic paraaortic metastases only. Welander *et al.* reported long-term survival in three of five patients (60%) with micrometastases, compared to five of 26 patients (19.2%) with gross paraaortic disease [36]. For the corresponding patient groups, Tewfik *et al.* reported survivals of 37.5% (three of eight) and 13.3% (two of fifteen) respectively [44]. Patients with gross involvement of paraaortic lymph nodes can usually be detected by a lymphangiogram and/or abdominal CT scan, and the diagnosis confirmed by fine needle aspiration cytology, thereby eliminating the need for surgical staging.

Unless the patients are being entered onto a research protocol, we presently restrict surgical staging to relatively young patients (premenopausal) who are in good general health, are not morbidly obese, and who have (1) a negative abdominal CT scan, and (2) stage IIA, IIB or unilateral IIIB disease. Patients with bulky stage IB disease would also be ideal candidates. In such patients, we obtain a pretreatment lymphangiogram and/or CT scan, and if positive paraaortic nodes are confirmed by fine needle aspiration cytology, extended field radiation is given. If the noninvasive tests are negative, we treat with pelvic radiation, and perform extrafascial hysterectomy 6 weeks postradiation, at which time we sample the paraaortic nodes, This avoids two operations, one for the surgical staging and the other for the hysterectomy. If positive nodes are found, an upper abdominal portal is added postoperatively.

The challenges for the future are to improve local tumor control in the pelvis and to develop effective systemic agents for metastatic cervical cancer. With the use of interstitial radiation techniques and/or chemoradiation, improved local tumor control may soon be a realistic expectation. If so, surgical staging will assume wider application until such time as more sensitive noninvasive tests are available for detecting paraaortic lymph node metastases.

References

1. Deppe G, Lubicz S, Galloway BT *et al.* 1984. Aortic node metastases with negative pelvic nodes in cervical cancer. Cancer 53:173.
2. Lifshitz SG, Buchsbaum HJ. 1977. The spread of cervical carcinoma. obstet Gynecol Ann 6:341.
3. Rutledge FN, Fletcher GH, MacDonald EJ. 1965. Pelvic lymphadenectomy as an adjunct to radiation therapy in treatment for cancer of the cervix. Am J Roentgenol 93:607.
4. Lagasse LD, Smith ML, Moore JG *et al.* 1974. The effect of radiation therapy on pelvic lymph node involvement in stage I carcinoma of the cervix. Am J Obstet Gynecol 119:328.
5. Koehler PR. 1976. Current status of lymphography in patients with cancer. Cancer 37:503.

6. Lecart C, Lenfant P. 1971. Criticial appraisal of lymphangiography in cancer of the female genital tract. Lymphology 3:100.
7. Wallace S, Jing BS, Zornoza J. 1977. Lymphangiography in the determination of extent of metastatic carcinoma. Cancer 39:706–718.
8. Piver SM, Barlow JJ. 1973. Para-aortic lymphadenectomy, aortic node biopsy, and aortic lymphangiography in staging patients with advanced cervical cancer. Cancer 32:367.
9. Littman P, Davis IW, Lepanto P. 1973. Evaluation of nodal metastases in patients with cervical carcinoma. Cancer 31:1307.
10. Brown RC. Buchsbaum HF, Tewfik HH, Platz CE. 1979. Accuracy of lymphangiography in the diagnosis of paraaortic lymph node metastases from carcinoma of the cervix. Obstet Gynecol 54:571.
11. Lagasse LD, Ballon SC, Berman ML, Watring WG. 1979. Pretreatment lymphangiography and the operative evaluation in carcinoma of the cervix. Am J Obstet Gynecol 134:219.
12. Kilcheski TS, Arger PH, Mulhern CB *et al.* 1981. Role of computed tomography in the presurgical evaluation of carcinoma of the cervix. J Comp Assist Tomogr 5:378.
13. Ginaldi S, Wallace S, King BS, Bernadino ME. 1981. Carcinoma of the cervix: lymphangiography and computed tomography. Am J Roentgenol 136:1087.
14. Photopulos GJ, McCartney WH, Walton LA, Staab EV. 1979. Computerized tomography applied to gynecologic ancology. Am J Obstet Gynecol. 135:381.
15. Brenner DE, Whitley NO, Prempree T, Villasanta U. 1982. An evaluation of the computed tomographic scanner for the staging of carcinoma of the cervix. Cancer 50:2323.
16. Whitley NO, Brenner DE, Francis A, Villasanta U, Aisher J, Wiernik PH, Whitley J. 1982. Computed tomographic evaluation of carcinoma of the cervix. Radiology 142:439.
17. Villasanta U, Whitley NO, Haney PJ, Brenner D. 1983. Computed tomography in invasive carcinoma of the cervix: An appraisal. Obstet Gynecol 62:218.
18. Bandy LC, Clarke-Pearson DL, Silverman P, Creasman WT. 1985. Computed Tomography in evaluation of extrapelvic lymphadenopathy in carcinoma of the cervix. Obstet Gynecol 65:73.
19. Lee JKT, Stanley RJ, Sagel SS, McClennan BL. 1978. Accuracy of CT in detecting intraabdominal and pelvic lymph node metastases from pelvic cancers. Am J Roentgenol 131:675.
20. Sommer FG, Walsh JW, Schwartz PE *et al.* 1982. Evaluation of gynecologic pelvic masses by ultrasound and computed tomography. J Reprod Med 27:45.
21. Moldofsky PJ, Sears HF, Mulhern CB *et al.* 1984. Detection of metastatic tumor in normal-sized retroperitoneal lymph nodes by monoclonal-antibody imaging. New Engl J Med 311:106.
22. Bies JR, Ellis JH, Kopecky KK *et al.* 1984. Assessment of primary gynecologic malignancies: comparison of 0.15-T resistive MRI with CT. Am J Roentgenol 143:1249.
23. Gothlin JH. 1976. Post-lymphangiographic fine needle biopsy of lymph nodes guided by fluoroscopy. Radiology 120:205.
24. McDonald TW, Morley GW, Choo YC *et al.* 1983. Fine needle aspiration of paraaortic and pelvic lymph nodes showing lymphangiographic abnormalities. Obstet Gynecol 61:383.
25. Zornosa J, Jonsson K, Wallace S *et al.* 1977. Fine needle aspiration biopsy of retroperitoneal lymph nodes and abdominal masses: An updated report. Radiology 125:87.
26. Berman ML, Lagasse LD, Watring WG *et al.* 1977. The operative evaluation of patients with cervical carcinoma by an extraperitoneal approach. Obstet Gynecol 50:658.
27. Delgado G, Chun B, Caglar H, Bepko F: 1977. Paraaortic lymphadenectomy in gynecologic malignancies confined to the pelvis. Obstet Gynecol 50:418.
28. Lagasse LD, Creasman WT, Shingleton HM *et al.* 1980. Results and complications of operative staging in cervical cancer: Experience of the Gynecologic Oncology Group. Gynecol Oncol 9:90.

29. Sudarsanem A, Charyulu K, Belinson J *et al.* 1978. Influence of exploratory celiotomy on the management of carcinoma of the cervix. Cancer 41:1049.
30. Nelson JH Jr, Boyce J, Masasaet M *et al.* 1977. Incidence, significance and follow-up of para-aortic lymph node metastases in late invasion carcinoma of the cervix. Am J Obstet Gynecol 128:336.
31. Wharton JT, Jones HW III, Day TG Jr *et al.* 1977. Preirradiation celiotomy and extended field irradiation for invasive carcinoma of the cervix. Obstet Gynecol 49:333.
32. Piver MS, Barlow JJ. 1977. High dose irradiation to biopsy confirmed aortic node metastases from carcinoma of the uterine cervix. Cancer 39:1243.
33. Buchsbaum HJ. 1979. Extrapelvic lymph node metastases in cervical carcinoma. Am J Obstet Gynecol 133:814.
34. Hughes RR, Brewington KC, Hanjani P *et al.* 1980. Extended field irradiation for cervical cancer based on surgical staging. gynecol Oncol 9:153.
35. Ballon SC, Berman ML, Lagasse LD *et al.* 1981. Survival after extraperitoneal pelvic and para-aortic lymphadenectomy and radiation therapy in cervical carcinoma. Obstet Gynecol 57:90.
36. Welander CE, Pierce VK, Nori D *et al.* 1981. Pretreatment laparotomy in carcinoma of the cervix. Gynecol Oncol 12:336.
37. Berman ML, Keys H, Creasman WT *et al.* 1984. Survival and patterns of recurrence in cervical cancer metastatic to periaortic lymph nodes. (A Gynecologic Oncology Group Study). Gynecol Oncol 19:8.
38. Potish RA, Twiggs LB, Okagaki T *et al.* 1985. Theurapeutic implications of the natural history of advanced cervical cancer as defined by pretreatment surgical staging. Cancer 56:956.
39. Goldson AL, Delgado G, Lawrence LT. 1978. Intraoperative radiation of the paraaortic nodes in cancer of the uterine cervix. Obstet Gynecol 52:713.
40. Potish R, Adcock L, Jones T Jr *et al.* 1983. The morbidity and utility of periaortic radiotherapy in cervical carcinoma. Gynecol Oncol 15:1.
41. El Senoussi MA, Fletcher GH, Borlase BC. 1979. Correlation of radiation and surgical parameters in complications in the extended field technique for carcinoma of the cervix. Int J Rad Oncol Biol Phys 5:927.
42. Piver MS, Barlow JJ, Krishnamsetty R. 1981. Five-year survival (with no evidence of disease) in patients with biopsy-confirmed aortic node metastases from cervical carcinoma. Am J Obstet Gynecol 139:575.
43. Rubin SC, Brookland R, Mikuta JJ *et al.* 1984. Paraaortic nodal metastases in early cervical carcinoma: long term survival following extended-field radiotherapy. Gynecol Oncol 18:213.
44. Tewfik HH, Buchsbaum HJ, Lafourette HB *et al.* 1982. Paraaortic lymph node irradiation in carcinoma of the cervix after exploratory laparotomy and biopsy-proven positive aortic nodes. Int J Rad Oncol Biol Phys 8:13.

5. Pre-operative radiotherapy for carcinoma of the cervix

NINA EINHORN

Introduction

Combined therapy of irradiation and surgery in the treatment of carcinoma of the cervix has been used in different ways for decades. The advocates of this combination offer explanations for the benetifs of combined therapy. These depend on whether they themselves are surgeons or radio therapists. The surgeons explain the advantages of pre-operative radiation as being the destruction of the primary neoplastic lesion, particularly at the edges of the tumour mass, decreasing the tumour cell spread during the operation. In addition they can make less extensive ureteral dissection, smaller vaginal cuffs as well as decreasing the surgical difficulties by reduction of the size of the tumour.

The arguments for adding surgery to irradiation are based on the recognition of radiation resistence in about 10% of the cases treated [1, 2]. Increased radioresistance as well as a risk for local recurrences recognized in younger women makes the combined approach particular applicable to these patients. In addition the possibility of giving postoperative irradiation complementary to lymphadenectomy in cases with bulky lymph node metastases is possible with the approach. An additional risk in younger women is that of developing a late secondary malignancy in the target organ [3].

There are very few randomized prospective studies comparing surgery or radiotherapy alone with the combined therapy. Rutledge and co-workers report a randomized study comparing lymphadenectomy after full course radiotherapy with radiotherapy alone [4]. A randomized prospective study was performed in Nairobi, East Africa, where combined therapy was compared with surgery alone [5]. None of these randomized studies gives a complete answer to the question of whether combined radiotherapy is better than either surgery or radiotherapy alone in the early cases and the answer to this question can only be found in the many publications of the findings in retrospective studies.

E.A. Surwit, D.S. Alberts (eds) Cervix Cancer.

Survival rates

As early as the 1930s and 1940s Leveuf [6] and Taussig [7] reported the results of pelvic lymphadenectomy following primary irradiation therapy. This was based on the recognized incidence of early metastases to regional pelvic lymph nodes and the premice that combined local and external irradiation is usually effective in controlling the primary lesion but not always effective for lymph node metastases. In 1943 Taussig reported a 38.6% 5-year survival in 70 patients with stage II lesions treated with complementary lymphadenectomy and compared these results with a 22.9% survival rate in a comparable series of 180 patients without lymphadenectomy [7]. Gordon was another advocate of lymphadenectomy following primary radiotherapy. In his collected data of combined therapy with intracavitary irradiation and lymphadenectomy alone, the survival rate for stage I lesions was essentially the same as that following radiation and surgery alone; with stage II lesions Gordon's results with combined therapy are significantly better than with radiotherapy or surgical therapy alone [8]. However, it was apparent that these treatment measures could not be used for all patients since evidence of control of the primary lesion by irradiation was a prerequisite for lymph node excision. Therefore it was only logical that other investigators frustrated by the prospect of cervical recurrence after lymphadenectomy extended the scope of complementary surgical therapy to include a radical hysterectomy.

Stallworthy was the first who in a consequent manner combined preoperative intracavitary treatment with radical surgery. In 1963 he explained the benefits of combined therapy by saying: 'It seems logical that if the primary growth was irradiated by a lethal tumour dose prior to operation there should be neither dissemination nor implantation of the viable cells. If the uterus, parameteria and adnexae were then removed, recurrent tumour formation could not occur in sites commonly involved following irradiation alone. A study of the exstirpated material was expected to throw light on the effects of irradiation therapy in the gynaecological tract and possibly help explain the reasons for local recurrence. As bilateral lymphadenectomy removes malignant glands and establishes their site of origin, supplemental irradiation could be concentrated where it should be most effective'. Stallworthy's philosophy created a school of combination therapy in stages IB, IIA and occasionally IIB, where intracavitary treatment was given preoperatively according to either the Stockholm, Paris or Manchester techniques. Stallwarthy found that after the application of radium according to the Stockholm technique with 7,200 mg/h spread over 3 weeks with an estimated dose of 3,000 rads at point A, the operation approximately three weeks after the last radium application was little effected technically by the radiation treatment. In his hands the 5-year cure rate of all patients was raised considerably by the application of combined therapy [9].

In an analysis of the results of treatment of carcinoma of cervix at the Radiumhemmet between 1949–1957 two factors were observed to influence the outcome unfavourably:
1. age; the prognosis tends to be worse in young women;
2. recurrence and persistance of the tumour locally in the cervix.
These two factors were the main reasons which lead to the adoption of combined therapy at Radiumhemmet and in 1963 Kottmeier proposed combination therapy in stage IB and IIA of women under 40 years of age.

Radiotherapy was given according to the Stockholm technique with two intracavitary treatments using intrauterine and intravaginal sources and about 2,500 mg/h in the uterus and 4,000 mg/h in the vagina. Two applications were given with a 3-week interval. Surgery was performed 4 weeks after the last intracavitary application. In most of the cases, if positive lymph nodes were found, external post-operative irradiation was added.

The results of this first series treated from 1963–1966 were evaluated in 1969 and at that time a decision was made to stop this treatment method partly because of the observed increased incidence of fistulas of the urinary tract. Cullhed later reported the survival rates of these patients; 168 women in stage IB and IIA were treated by combined treatment with preoperative radiation therapy and radical hysterectomy; 621 women in the same stages were treated by radiotherapy alone. The 5-year survival rate for the combined group and radiotherapy only group for stage IB was 89.9 and 83.5% respectively, and for stage IIA 76.8 and 62.3% respectively [10]. Between 1969–1972 all patients at Radiumhemmet were treated with radiotherapy alone. As an increased recurrence rate locally in younger women was again observed, from 1972 the combined treatment modality was once again applied to all patients in stage IB and IIA younger than 40 years. These very distinct periods of time with different approaches to therapy allow one to make comparisons of unselected series of cases of younger women who received either preoperative irradiation and radical surgery or radiotherapy alone. The results show a significant difference in survival for stage IB giving 96% 5-year survival rate for the combined group and 81% for radiotherapy alone. No significant difference could be seen in stage IIA disease which gave a 74% survival rate for radiotherapy alone and a 66% survival rate in the combined treatment group [11].

Similar results have been reported from another Swedish clinic in Gothenburg where patients were treated with or without surgery depending on age. For these two groups treated during the years 1970–1977 the 5-year survival rate for radiotherapy alone was 85% and for the group receiving combined therapy 90% in stage IB and for stage IIA the survival rate for the two treatment groups was 70 and 77% respectively [12]. In Oslo during the years 1967–1972 147 patients in stage IB were treated with radiotherapy alone and 562 underwent combined treatment. The results showed a 5-year survival rate of 84% for the combined group and 71% for those receiving radiotherapy only [13].

In Southern Sweden two clinics with different approaches to treatment of stage IB disease compared their results. The Malmoe clinic treated patients with combined treatment and the survival rate rate in a series of 221 cases with stage IB disease was 88%. The results for stage IB patients treated with radiotherapy alone at the University Clinic of Lund show a 5-year survival rate of 91%. However, the combined treatment gave better results in women younger than 35 years of age giving a survival rate of 93% in the combined group of Malmoe hospital and an 81% survival rate in the radiotherapy group of Lund's hospital.

Surwit and co-workers performed a retrospective study to evaluate the effectivenss of preoperative irradiation by comparing patients in stage IB treated by surgery alone with patients treated with combination therapy. The 5-year crude survival rate for the combined group was 89.7% and for patients treated with surgery alone 75.1% [15].

Residual tumour

Several reports confirm that the finding of residual tumour in the surgical specimen can be correlated to the prognosis. In Villasanta's series of combined therapy the 5-year survival rate for patients with residual disease was 61 versus 95% in those with no residual tumour [16]. In Mogens Kern Hansen's series from Denmark residual tumour in the cervix was associated with an increased incidence of lymph node metastases and a poorer prognosis [17]. In Marziale's series of combined radiation and surgical treatment in stage IB and IIA better results were obtained when no residual tumour was found; 86.8 versus 54.3% [18]. In the Oslo series presented by Rampone and co-workers 7.2% of the patients with pelvic or vaginal recurrence had residual cancer in the hysterectomy specimen [2]. In Lloy D. Bonar's series the presence of residual tumour decreased the 5-year survival rate from 93.4 to 61.0% [19]. Even in the latest series of Timmer and co-workers the presence of residual tumour showed a high correlation to the presence of lymph node metastases and both together were the most significant prognostic factors. Among the patients with residual tumour, 43% has lymph node metastases [20]. In the Stockholm series the presence of residual tumour had no impact on the survival in stage IB but in stage IIA 38% of the patients with residual tumour had died of their disease [11].

Complications

The risk of an increased complication rate has been the argument most used against combination therapy. With a better understanding of the problems associated with combining radiotherapy and surgery a less radical surgical approach has emerged, less extensive ureteral dissection has been one factor in decreasing the rate of complications using combined therapy during the years.

Novak in 1963 analyzed the causes of fistula in his surgical series and pointed out that one has to take three precautions to decrease the incidence of fistulas, sparing the tissue lateral to the points at which the ureters enter the bladder, division of the uterine arteries late in the operation and securing the ureters intraperitoneally. He succeeded in reducing the incidence of fistulae from 11.4 to 2.8% during the period 1954–1962 [21]. In the Stockholm series the importance of not removing the periureteral tissue clearly explain the difference in complication rate. During the years 1963–1966 three clinics were participating in the surgery after pre-operative irradiation. In principal two of them followed the Meigs technique and in the third one all periureteral tissue at the junction of ureters and bladder was removed. At the two first clinics the percentage of fistulas was 2.8% and at the third one 17.3% [10]. In the later series when less radical dissection around the ureters was performed the incidence of ureteral complications dropped to 0 and bowel complications to 1.3% [11]. Table 1 illustrates the percentages of fistulas in the latest published series of patients treated with combined therapy.

Conclusions

Pre-operative irradiation can be safely given to stages IB and IIA carcinoma of the cervix , the aim being to treat the local cervical tumor and destroy it

Table 1.

	Ureteral fistulas (%)	Bowel complications (%)
Marziale (1981) [18]	1.8	
Surwit (1976) [15]	5.0	2.0
De Graaff (1980)	2.9	2.9
Rampone (1973) [2]	2.8	
Weed (1977)	1.9	
Bonar (1980) [19]	4.2	1.0
Timmer (1984) [20]	2.0	1.5
Einhorn (1985) [11]	0	1.3

totally, if possible. The pre-operative irradiation diminishes the risk of cancer cell spread during surgery, allowing a shorter vaginal cuff and makes the surgical procedure less difficult.

Surgery after pre-operative irradiation removes the possibility of local tumour recurrence, indicates the location of lymph node metastases to best define postoperative irradiation if indicated. In younger women it eliminates the risk of developing late secondary malignancies in the heavily irradiated target organ.

References

1. Kottmeier H-L. 1964. Surgical and radiation treatment of carcinoma of the uterine cervix. Acta Obstet Gynecol Scand 43 (Suppl 2): 1–48.
2. Rampone JF, Klem V, Kolstad P. 1973. Combined treatment of stage IB carcinoma of the cervix. Obstet Gynecol 41: 163–167.
3. Pettersson F, Foriou S, Einhorn N, Silfverswärd C. 1985. Cohort study of the long-term effect of irradiation for carcinoma of the uterine cervix. Acta Radiol Oncol Fasc 224: 145–151.
4. Rutledge FN, Fletcher GH, MacDonald EE. 1965. Pelvic lymphadenectomy as an adjunct to radiation therapy in treatment for cancer of the cervix. Am J Roentgenol Radium Ther Nucl Med 93: 607–614.
5. Einhorn N, Einhorn L, Gebbie DAM, Willey B. 1974. Preoperative radiotherapy in the treatment of cervical carcinoma in Africa. XI International Cancer Congress in Florence.
6. Leveuf J, Godard H. 1934. L'envahissement des ganglions lymphatiques dans le cancer du col de l'uterus. J Chir (Paris) 43: 177.
7. Taussig FJ. 1943. Iliac lymphadenectomy for group II cancer of the cervix. Am J Obstet Gynecol 45: 733–748.
8. Gordon G. 1957. Radiation therapy and excision of the lymph nodes in cervical cancer. Progr Gynecol 3: 594–603.
9. Stallworthy J. 1964. Radical surgery following radiation treatment for cervical carcinoma. Ann Roy College Surg Engl 34: 161–178.
10. Cullhed S. 1978. Carcinoma cervicis uteri stages I and IIA. Linköping University Medical Dissertation No. 59.
11. Einhorn N, Patek E, Sjöberg B. 1985. Outcome of different treatment modalities in cervix carcinoma stage IB and IIA. Cancer 55: 949–955.
12. Jansson I, Himmelmann A, Dennefors B, Bendz A. 1984. Results of combined rediological and surgical therapy of carcinoma of the uterine cervix stage IB and IIA (Abstract). Nordisk Forening for Obstetrik og gynaekologi, Odense, Denmark.
13. Iversen T, Kjöstad KE, Martimbeau PW. 1982. Treatment results in carcinoma of the cervix stage IB in a total population. Gynecol Oncol 14: 1–5.
14. Gynning I, Johnsson J-E, Alm P, Tropé C. 1983. Age and prognosis in stage IB squamous cell carcinoma of the uterine cervix. Gynecol Oncol 15: 18–26.
15. Surwit E, Fowler WC Jr, Palumbo L, Koch G, Gjertsen W. 1976. Radical hysterectomy with or without preoperative radium for stage IB squamous cell carcinoma of the cervix. Obstet Gynecol 48: 130–133.
16. Villasanta U. 1967. Combined radium therapy and radical hysterectomy with pelvic lymphadenectomy in treatment of invasive cancer of the cervix. Obst Gyrecol 32: 6–10.
17. Hansen MK. 1981. Surgical and combination therapy of cancer of the cervix of the cervix uteri stages IB and IIA. Gynecol Oncol 11: 275–287.

18. Marziale P, Atlante V, Le Pera V, Marino T, Pozzi M, Iacovelli A. 1981. Combined radiation and surgical treatment of stages IB and IIA carcinoma of the cervix. Gynecol Oncol 11:175–183.
19. Bonar LD. 1980. Results of radical surgical procedures after radiation for treatment of invasive carcinoma of the uterine cervix in a private practice. Am J Obstet Gynecol 136:1006–1008.
20. Timmer PR, Aalders HG, Bouma J. 1984. Radical surgery after preoperative intracavitary radiotherapy for stage IB and IIA carcinoma of the uterine cervix. Gynecol Oncol 18:206–212.
21. Novak F. 1963. Procedure for the reduction of the number of ureterovaginal fistulas after Wertheim's operation. Proc R Soc Med 56:881.

6. Radical hysterectomy and pelvic lymphadenectomy

KARL C. PODRATZ and RICHARD E. SYMMONDS

Introduction

The advent of the twentieth century witnessed the initiation of radical abdominal surgery for the treatment of uterine cancers. Recognizing the pattern of direct infiltrative extension and nodal metastases, Wertheim [1] championed an extirpative procedure that included wide parametrial resections with ureteral mobilization, inclusion of an extended segment of the uterosacral ligaments, and excision of a generous portion of the vagina and sampling of suspicious pelvic nodes. Wertheim's experience with 500 cases included an operative mortality of 18% which was predominantly attributable to the difficulties in managing postoperative infections. Because of the associated operative mortality and the evolving applications of radiotherapy, enthusiasm for the surgical treatment of cervical carcinoma was nearly dormant for several decades.

Medical advances in blood grouping and antimicrobial therapy aided the renaissance of radical pelvic surgery, which was pioneered by Meigs [2] in this country approximately 45 years ago. Recognizing the significance of occult carcinomatous involvement of palpably normal lymph nodes, Meigs expanded the Wertheim operation by including a formal pelvic lymphadenectomy and a more complete removal of the parametrium. He reported his personal experience through 1946, stating, 'with careful surgery and the use of sulfonamides and antibiotics, 100 patients were operated upon with no hospital mortality' [3]. In addition, the therapeutic results were equally impressive and compared favorably with the results obtained with radiotherapy by his contemporaries and, hence, rekindled enthusiasm for this surgical approach, both nationally and internationally.

The subsequent evolution of radical hysterectomy and pelvic lymphadenectomy for the treatment of cervical carcinoma included definition of the indications and limitations of this surgical approach and assessment of the etiologic factors leading to and curtailment of surgical morbidity. During the

E.A. Surwit, D.S. Alberts (eds) Cervix Cancer.
 ISBN 0-89838-822-8. Printed in the Netherlands.

past four decades numerous reports have described institutional experience with this procedure, collectively establishing its efficacy in the treatment of locally infiltrative disease. Several groups have prospectively compared radical hysterectomy and pelvic radiotherapy and, based on patient survivorship, demonstrated similar therapeutic benefits [4–6]. In addition, various modifications have been incorporated with the intent of diminishing postoperative morbidity; these have included alterations in techniques to minimize associated urinary complications. Nevertheless, the radical hysterectomy and lymphadenectomy as performed at this institution and described below remains largely unaltered in principle from the traditional Wertheim-Meigs procedure.

Indications and pre-operative evaluation

The selection of a surgical approach in the treatment of any oncologic process should include demonstrable benefit compared with alternate noninvasive modalities, definition of the indications and limitations of the procedure, and identification of contraindications to its use. Although anatomic and physiologic alterations accompany both the radiologic and surgical treatment of invasive cervical carcinoma, the latter provides several advantages. Surgery allows the option of preserving ovarian function. This consideration has become of increasing importance as the mean age at menopause has increased and the median age at diagnosis of cervical cancer has decreased. Furthermore, although the vagina is foreshortened, the tissue integrity and organ functionality are generally superior after radical hysterectomy than in the postirradiated vagina. Similarly, long-term bowel and bladder effects resulting from tissue fibrosis and endarteritic obliteration which accompany whole pelvic irradiation are avoided with operation. In addition, with the deficiencies inherent in clinical staging [7], operation affords a definitive evaluation of the extent of neoplastic involvement and, in conjunction with pathologic evaluation, provides the basis for more precise individual prognostication and planning of adjuvant therapy.

The clinical extent of disease and various demographic characteristics have formed the basis for surgical eligibility at most institutions. With rare exceptions, patients presenting with stage IB 'occult', IB, or IIA squamous cell carcinoma of the cervix are treated with radical hysterectomy and pelvic lymphadenectomy at our clinic. The same surgical approach is used in treating these early invasive lesions when they are associated with pregnancy, when they originate in a cervical stump, or when they are identified in a specimen after a simple hysterectomy. Although concern over enhanced blood loss during pregnancy usually exists, cleavage planes and vascular tributaries are readily identified and, therefore, frequently facilitate the dissection. In contrast, radical trachelectomy and radical reoperation after simple hysterectomy are technically more challenging in that the usual traction and countertraction vectors are altered in the absence of the uterine corpus. Adenocarcinomas of either primary cervical origin or extension from the endometrium are considered therapeutically amenable to the same type of radical uterine extirpation. In addition, the persistence of carcinoma localized to the cervix after completion of primary pelvic irradiation is an additional indication for this procedure. The patient and physician must recognize and accept the additional morbidity that is associated with this sequence of therapy. Furthermore, previous experience with managing post-irradiation persistent disease that penetrated the endopelvic fascia and required an 'extended' Wertheim-Meigs procedure (either partial bladder, ureteral, or rectosigmoid resection) demonstrated an appreciable complication rate [8, 9]. Therefore, more liberal use of exenterative procedures with neovaginal reconstruction is appropriate and also affords more generous margins of clearance which potentially extrapolate to improved long-term prognosis.

With rare exceptions, patients with relative contraindications, including those with significant medical conditions and the geriatric subset (age > 65 years), can be adequately prepared to tolerate the moderate anesthetic and surgical stresses associated with this procedure. A detailed history and physical examination, including clinical assessment of the pelvis for clinical staging purposes, comprise the essentials of the preanesthetic medical evaluation (PAME). Laboratory analyses necessary to complete the PAME include electrocardiography, chest radiography, excretory urography, hematologic values, serum chemistries, urinalysis, and coagulation profile. Thereafter, detectable alterations in normal physiologic functions require expeditious clinical investigation and prompt correction. Cytoscopy, proctoscopy, radiologic imaging of the gastrointestinal tract, computed axial tomography, sonography, and lymphangiography can, on occasion, provide additional pre–operative information that is justifiable from a cost-benefit standpoint only when used on a highly selective basis. In addition, cervical conization is frequently used to differentiate stages IA and IB prior to initiating definitive therapy. The associated morbidity, as reflected in complications following hysterectomy after conization and the appropriate time interval between these two procedures, has been debated [10–13]. The distance to referral sites and the associated inconveniences have generally not allowed the option of selecting an 'ideal' interval separating conization and radical hysterectomy at our institution. A recent evaluation failed to show correlations among prehysterectomy conization or various intervening time intervals and additional febrile morbidity, wound infections, pelvic abscesses, or technical difficulties in executing the hysterectomy [13].

Operative technique

Exploration

An incision should be chosen that will conveniently allow the anticipated completion of the operative procedure and not compromise access to the periaortic area or upper abdominal viscera if circumstances dictate extension of the primary operation or necessitate inclusion of a secondary procedure. The authors prefer a lower midline incision, skirting the umbilicus, that can be extended cephalad with ease when indicated. On entry into the abdominal cavity, peritoneal fluid or washings of pelvic viscera are routinely obtained for cytologic evaluation. Systematic evaluation of all abdominal viscera, including the internal genitalia, is stressed; on occasion this reveals additional pathology potentially requiring concomitant surgical treatment. The periaortic node-bearing regions are initially examined from pelvic brim to the diaphragm with sampling of all palpably suspicious nodes. Based on the extent and location of periaortic involvement, the operative procedure may be terminated if extensive nodal disease is encountered (rarely observed in clinical stage IB and IIA patients). When distal periaortic and caval nodal metastases are noted, the authors prefer to complete a formal periaortic node dissection. This is also performed when metastatic common iliac adenopathy is identified, as described below. After completion of the exploration, the patient is placed in an exaggerated Trendelenburg position ($\geq 45°$ angle), which facilitates gravitational venous return from the lower extremities and minimizes the amount of packing of extrapelvic viscera at the pelvic brim, which in turn avoids venous compression and additional venous stasis.

Development of paravesical and pararectal spaces

Although ideal exposure is preferable during any surgical procedure, the anatomic constraints inherent in the pelvis require complete familiarity with the various true and potential tissue spaces and their relation to adjacent structures as well as an appreciation of proper traction and countertraction forces to maximize exposure. The development of the pararectal and paravesical spaces (Figure 1) facilitates the expeditious completion of the pelvic lymphadenectomy and the radical hysterectomy. The round ligament is transected and the peritoneum is incised in a superior fashion along the ovarian vessels and inferiorly toward the vesicouterine peritoneal reflection. Lateral retraction of the ligated round ligament and firm medial traction of the uterine corpus expose the anterior planes of the pararectal and paravesical spaces. The anatomic landmarks for the former include the pelvic ureter

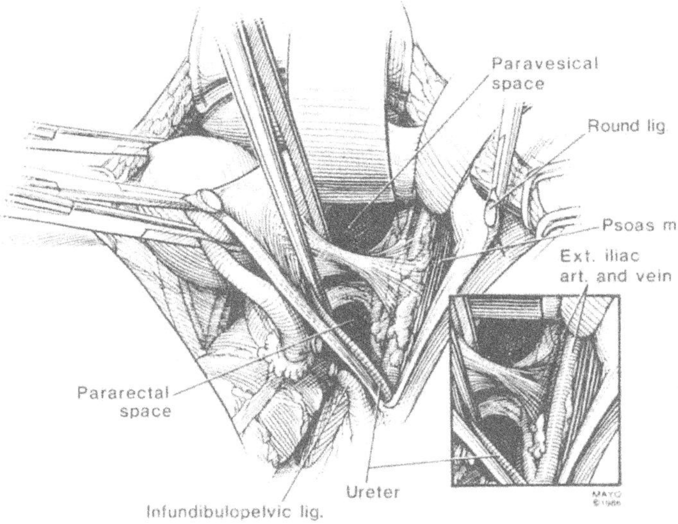

Figure 1. Contralateral traction of uterine corpus and development of pararectal and paravesical spaces provide access to lateral pelvic web and pelvic lymph node-bearing tissues (by permission of Mayo Foundation).

medially and the internal iliac artery laterally. Separation of these structures and continued blunt dissection of the avascular areolar tissue in a posterior and slightly medial direction develops the pararectal space, exposing the major portion of the pelvic ureter attached to the peritoneum, the internal iliac vessels and accompanying lymphatic tissue, and the superior border of the lateral pelvic web.

The anatomic landmarks for entry into the paravesical space include the external iliac artery laterally and the obliterated umbilical artery medially. Posterior and inferior blunt dissection through the avascular areolar tissue continues until the fascia overlying the pelvic floor is exposed. This dissection defines the inferior border of the lateral pelvic web and allows ready access to the obturator fossa. The placement of a wide Deaver retractor (Figure 1) in the perivesical space for anterior and inferior soft-tissue displacement provides generous exposure during subsequent lymphatic dissection and ligation of the lateral pelvic web.

The authors emphasize that ureteral or bladder dissection or mobilization is delayed until near the terminal phases of the procedure. This delay eliminates the need for prolonged displacement and retraction of the ureters, thereby decreasing ureteral ischemia and dehydration. Furthermore, the transection of the vascular vesicouterine web for ureteral mobilization is also delayed, deferring a potential source of blood loss until near the end of the procedure.

Pelvic lymphadenectomy

With rare exceptions, in patients presenting with clinical stage IB and IIA lesions, the authors attempt to accomplish a formal pelvic lymphadenectomy even in the presence of surgically or histologically apparent metastatic nodal involvement. Circumstances suggesting abandonment of the procedure have been referred to above and pertain to extensive periaortic disease. Our inclusion of a complete periaortic node dissection is dependent on the finding of positive proximal pelvic (common iliac) nodes. This approach is aided by the availability at our institution of immediate histologic assessment of all removed lymph nodes via frozen section.

The lymphadenectomy begins with removal of the perivascular soft-tissue matrix from the external iliac artery. With a wide Deaver retractor in the paravesical space and a narrow Deaver retractor directed along the axis of the vessels and retracted anteriorly and distally, the inferior epigastric vessels (and infrequently the deep circumflex vessels) are readily identified and the soft-tissue matrix is dissected from the anterior, medial, and lateral aspects of the external iliac vessels. This lymphatic pad is elevated with a thumb forceps and swept cephalad with a dissecting shears until the bifurcation of the common iliac artery is encountered. The wide Deaver retractor is repositioned and used to retract the ovarian vessels, ureter, and medial peritoneum in a superior and medial fashion while the repositioned narrow Deaver retracts the lateral peritoneum superiorly and laterally, exposing the common iliac vessels, inferior vena cava, and aorta. The bifurcation of the aorta identifies the superior margin of the pelvic lymphadenectomy. The soft-tissue matrix is interrupted at this point and meticulously elevated and mobilized toward the bifurcation of the common iliac vessels. Frequently, small perforating veins are encountered entering the lymphatic pad from the vena cava and common iliac vein and are divided by hemoclips. If these veins are inadvertently transected, the accompanying bleeding can be managed with gentle tamponade by interfacing a surgical sponge between the bleeding point and the overlying peritoneum or soft tissues. The presacral and internal iliac node dissection is completed while exposure is optimal at this point.

The obturator node dissection is initiated by retracting the psoas muscle laterally with the narrow Deaver and mobilizing the common iliac vessels medially (Figure 2). Removal of the soft-tissue matrix beneath and lateral to the common iliac vessels exposes the obturator nerve, lumbosacral trunk, and venous branches forming the major tributaries of the internal iliac vein. The lymphatic pad is mobilized along the lateral aspects of the iliac veins in an inferior fashion. After replacement of the wide Deaver in the paravesical space and retraction of the external iliac vessels laterally, the obturator node dissection continues in the obturator fossa. Cleansing the obturator fossa

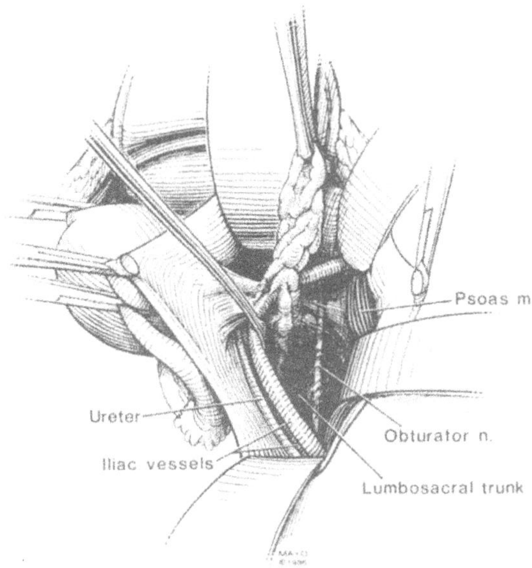

Figure 2. Lateral retraction of psoas muscle and medial displacement of common and proximal external iliac vessels facilitate dissection of proximal obturator lymphatic chain. Lumbosacral trunk, obturator nerve, and numerous parietal branches of the internal iliac vessels are identifiable (by permission of Mayo Foundation).

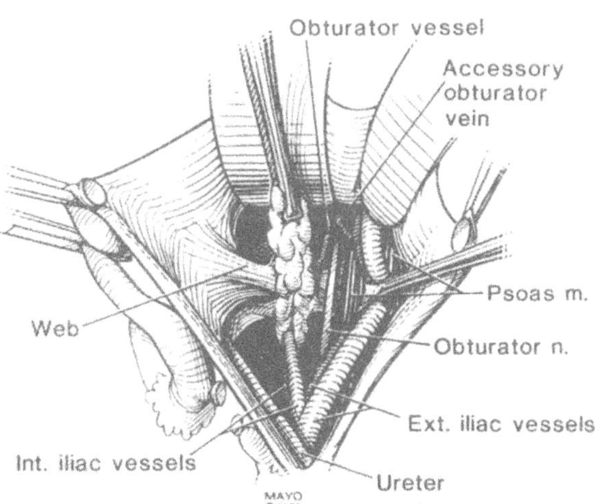

Figure 3. Obturator lymphadenectomy is completed with removal of loose tissue matrix in obturator fossa. Identification of obturator nerve, the more variable obturator and accessory obturator vessels, and rich venous network below obturator nerve minimizes vascular trauma and annoying blood loss (by permission of Mayo Foundation).

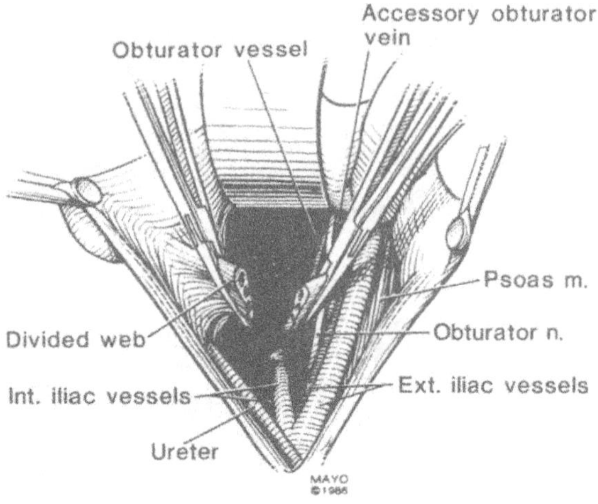

Figure 4. After blunt undermining of condensations of endopelvic fascia in posterior portion of lateral pelvic web, the web is doubly clamped, transected, and ligated near pelvic sidewall (by permission of Mayo Foundation).

requires identification of the obturator and accessory obturator vessels to avoid trauma and annoying bleeding. All soft tissue is removed, stripping obturator vessels and the nerve until the delicate venous network beneath these structures is adequately skeletonized (Figure 3). An entire hemipelvic lymphadenectomy can be accomplished in an *en bloc* fashion with minimal blood loss and pathologically evaluated while the node dissection on the contralateral side is performed.

Ligation of lateral pelvic web and uterosacral ligaments

Proper development of the perirectal and perivesical spaces as described above essentially skeletonizes the lateral pelvic web through which course branches of the internal iliac vessels, lymphatic channels, nerves to and from the central pelvic organs, and condensations of the endopelvic fascia. The anterior division of the internal iliac artery (and occasionally vein) is independently ligated, allowing more flexibility and ease of ligation of the lateral pelvic web. The posterior contents of the web are palpated and blunt passage of a digit through the loose tissue beneath the cardinal ligament allows parallel placement of long hemostats adjacent to the pelvic sidewall (Figure 4). A single ligature generally suffices, but in the irradiated pelvis, the hemostat is undersewn, removed, and the pedicle oversewn to assure adequate hemostasis. Significant bleeding is seldom encountered, but when inadvertent trauma to the generous venous network occurs, the authors

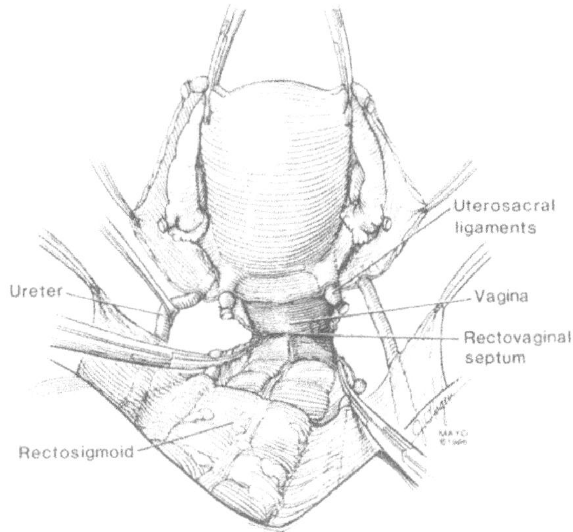

Figure 5. After mobilization of distal portions of pelvic ureters from pelvic peritoneum, the peritoneum is incised, allowing access into rectrovaginal septum for posterior displacement of rectosigmoid and ligation of uterosacral ligaments (by permission of Mayo Foundation).

avoid packing and prefer gentle digital tamponade, with undersewing of the digit apex and closure of the vascular defect as the digit is withdrawn. At least in part, bladder 'numbness' and dysfunction are reflections of the degree of radicality in the resection of the lateral pelvic web, and the authors occasionally tailor this portion of the resection if the lesion characteristics are clinically and surgically considered favorable.

After lateral interruption of the endopelvic fascial condensations, the uterine corpus is considerably more mobile, facilitating the subsequent dissection. The midportion of the pelvic ureters is separated from the peritoneum and the uterus is displaced anteriorly and inferiorly. With countertraction on the sigmoid, the peritoneum is incised (carefully avoiding the ureters), exposing the uterosacral ligaments and the potential rectovaginal space. The latter is developed under direct vision, using sharp dissection and continuous anterior traction of the genitalia and countertraction of the rectosigmoid. The posterior mobilization is completed with ligation of the uterosacral ligaments and the adjacent perirectal soft tissues (Figure 5).

Mobilization of bladder and ureters

In addition to minimizing trauma, ischemia, and drying, delaying the mobilization of the bladder and ureters until near the completion of the pro-

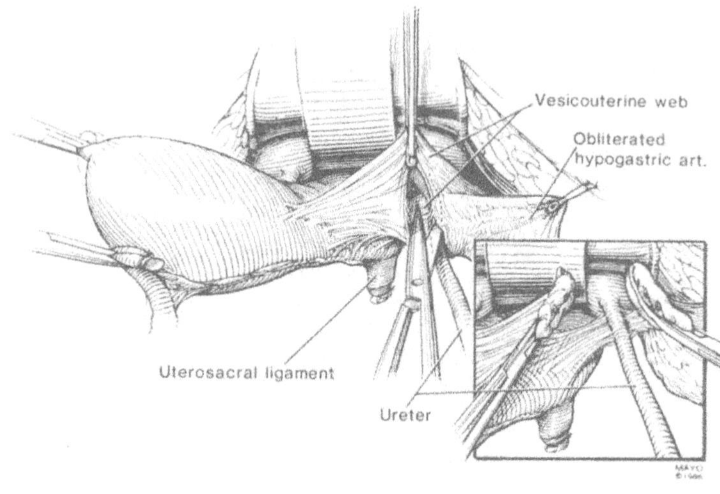

Figure 6. Inferior displacement of bladder, lateral retraction of transected obliterated umbilical artery, and countertraction of the uterine corpus create sufficient tension on vesicouterine web for ease of tunneling (under direct vision) of distal ureter and subsequent transection of anterior portion of vesicouterine web (by permission of Mayo Foundation).

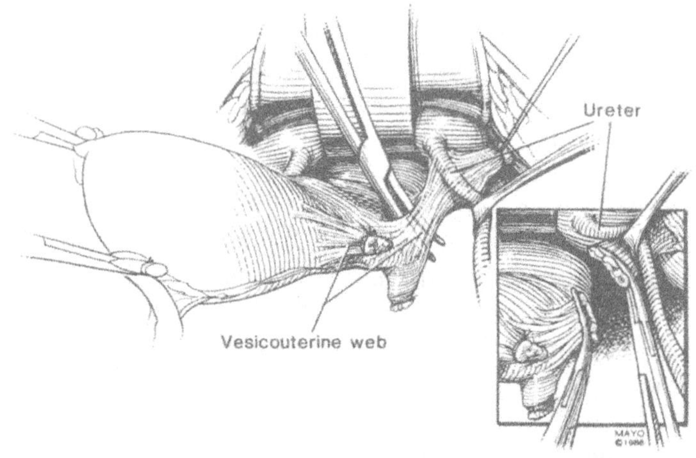

Figure 7. Posterior portion of vesicouterine web is isolated and transected, resulting in complete mobilization of distal collecting system (by permission of Mayo Foundation).

cedure greatly facilitates their dissection. Resection of the lateral pelvic webs and the uterosacral ligaments results in anterior and superior displacement of the uterus and vagina, allowing better access to the vesicovaginal septum and the vesicouterine webs. After incision of the vesicouterine peritoneum, sharp dissection is used to separate the bladder from the anterior aspect of the vagina, 1–2 cm below the anticipated point of vaginal transection. With displacement of the bladder inferiorly (using a wide Deaver or Harrington retractor) and the uterine corpus laterally and superiorly, the vesicouterine web is adequately displayed. After ligation of the obliterated hypogastric artery, the ureter is placed under gentle countertraction and tunneled free from beneath the anterior division of the vesicouterine web (Figure 6). The web is divided and ligated, resulting in complete unroofing of the distal ureter (Figure 6). Anterior displacement of the distal ureter allows access to the posterior division of the vesicouterine web which is interrupted (Figure 7). The lateral pedicle of the posterior division of the vesicouterine web serves as a tissue cradle for lateral displacement of the ureter for the duration of the procedure.

Management of the vagina and retroperitoneum

The endopelvic fascia encircling the vagina is circumferentially incised prior to transecting the vagina. Approximately 25% of the vagina is sacrificed with stage IB lesions, whereas a more extended partial vaginectomy, preferably 2–3 cm margins of clearance, is performed with stage IIA lesions. Prior to vaginal vault closure, the resected borders of the vagina should be histologically evaluated via frozen section. Primary vaginal cuff closure is accomplished in a two-layered fashion; an initial submucosal reapproximation is

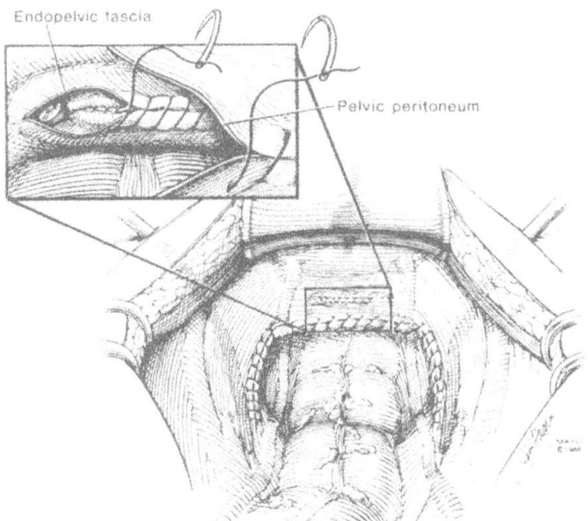

Figure 8. Vagina in closed in a two-layered fashion: mucosa to mucosa, followed by perivaginal fascia reapproximations. Reperitonealization is accomplished over vagina, ureters, and suction drains traversing obturator fossa. Ovaries, when preserved, are suspended near pelvic brim. Suprapubic cystostomy is preferred approach for securing adequate bladder drainage (by permission of Mayo Foundation).

followed by reapproximation of the previously incised perivaginal fascia (Figure 8). Without specific attention to ureteral location, pelvic reperitonealization is accomplished in a semilunar fashion, suspending the ovaries when preserved near the pelvic brim. Drains are dropped into the obturator fossa to provide suction evacuation of lymphatic fluid, blood, and debris, allowing rapid adherence of the peritoneum to the underlying structures (Figure 8). A suprapubic cystostomy is performed prior to closure of the abdominal incision.

Post–operative complications

Incision

Although wound infections were observed in approximately 6% of nonirradiated patients between 1955 and 1975 [9], it is estimated that this rate has decreased substantially during the past decade. The authors suspected that the routine incorporation in the abdominal incision closure of a subcutaneous catheter attached to either continuous or intermittent low suction for removal of serosanguineous debris for 3–4 days postoperatively, as suggested by McIlrath *et al.* [14], has been more influential in lowering the wound infection rate than 'prophylactic antibiotics'. The removal via this technique of small quantities of blood or serum which occasionally accumulate during the immediate postoperative phase essentially eliminates the natural *in situ* culture medium for various microbes. Once suspected, infected wounds are treated promptly by opening the incision beyond the margins of inflammation and generally down to the fascia, obtaining appropriate cultures for microbes in the process. Subsequent irrigation with water or saline, half-strength Dakin's solution, or diluted Betadine solution (avoid hydrogen peroxide) and open packing secures a granulation tissue base ideal for either secondary surgical or passive closure.

Retroperitoneum

Although pelvic abscesses are more prone to occur in previously irradiated patients, particularly those subjected to extended radical procedures, they are rarely encountered when the operative procedure described above constitutes primary therapy. Routine closure of the vaginal vault, pelvic reperitonealization, retroperitoneal suction catheter drainage [15], and meticulous hemostasis and liberal preclosure lavage minimize the source and size of the bacterial inoculum and the natural medium for bacterial proliferation. Nevertheless, on recognition of an abscess, prompt surgical management, including incision, debridement, and drainage via either a transvaginal or extraperitoneal approach, is indicated. The debridement of cavitary defects in heavily irradiated areas is aided by frequent pressurized pulsatile water irrigations and packing changes until cavitary closure is complete. However, definitive closure occasionally requires procurement of a more adequate blood supply. Our preference at present is the mobilization of the gracilis muscle and, when indicated, this may be accompanied by a cutaneous island.

Management of the pelvic retroperitoneum as described above also comprises preventative control of postoperative lymphocele formation [15]. Catheter aspiration of the surgically developed spaces continues until the 24-h aspirated volume is less than 50 ml for 2 consecutive days. The incidence of occult asymptomatic lymphocysts is difficult to ascertain but undoubtedly higher than appreciated, and spontaneous regression is commonplace. Asymptomatic, incidentally detected lymphocysts require expectant management only. Obstructive uropathy (usually secondary to an adynamic segment of ureter adjacent to the lymphocyst), infection (infrequent and managed as pelvic abscess), and persistent pain or significant lower extremity edema resulting from retroperitoneal accumulation of lymphatic fluid are indications for a secondary drainage procedure. Because of minimal associated morbidity, needle aspirations or imaging-directed percutaneous catheter placements are worthy of initial consideration. However, our experience with these methods, including sclerosing trials with tetracycline, has resulted in only meager success. Surgical excision of a portion of the medial wall of the lymphocyst and adjacent peritoneum, with or without omental transposition, is recommended in cases not responding to more conservative management.

Vascular

The natural and essentially avascular cleavage planes, including the pararectal and paravesical spaces and vesicovaginal and rectovaginal septa, facilitate dissection and minimize blood loss during the radical hysterectomy. When blood replacement is required, it is generally attributable to bleeding encountered during the pelvic lymphadenectomy and interruption of the vesicouterine web and, less frequently, to ligation of the lateral pelvic web. Deliberate or inadvertent transection of a small vein during lymphatic stripping seldom requires interruption of surgical rhythm (or hemoclip placement) but simply interfacing of a surgical sponge between the bleeding focus and the adjacent tissues, allowing gentle tissue tamponade. Although avulsions from and lacerations of major venous tributaries are uncommon, digital tamponade with meticulous repair of the defect by using vascular suture (i.e., 5–0 vascular silk) for undersewing at the apex of the surgeon finger as it is progressively withdrawn is recommended. It is preferable to avoid packs, which decrease venous return and enhance thrombotic events, or attempts at hemostat placement, which not infrequently result in extension of the vascular defect. With the above mangement, the majority of patients subjected to this procedure have required only one unit or no blood replacement at our institution [9].

Clinically perceptible thrombophlebitis occurred with a frequency of approximately 5% in our patient population [5]. Unless the pre-anesthetic medical evaluation identifies specific risk factors, prophylactic anticoagulants have not been routinely used. The authors' reluctance to use perioperative heparin is based on the potential increased operating interval from alterations in the approach secondary to hemostasis, increased volume and prolonged postoperative lymphatic drainage, increased rate of hematoma formation, and the accompanying enhanced morbidity from each of these sequelae. Clinical evidence consistent with the most significant sequelae of venous thrombosis, namely, pulmonary embolization, occurred once in every 53 patients, with one death occurring among 610 such cases [9]. However, necessity of maximizing venous return from the lower extremities and avoiding excessive large-vessel trauma are of utmost importance. Our practice includes (1) placing the patient in an exaggerated Trendelenburg position to allow enhanced gravitational venous return, (2) no operating table restraints except for special ankle straps, (3) minimal pressure from abdominal pack over distal inferior vena cava or common iliac vessels, (4) elastic support stockings to aid uniform support of soft tissue in the lower extremities, (5) expeditious operation, thereby avoiding prolonged operating times, (6) early postoperative ambulation, and (7) minimal manipulation (particularly for controlling bleeding) of major pelvic venous tributaries.

Whereas the internal iliac artery and its numerous branches can be sacrificed without appreciable sequelae, significant trauma to the aorta and common and external iliac arteries must be recognized and corrected to avoid compromise of function of the lower extremities. Partial or complete transection of these vessels requires adequate mobilization and occlusion above and below the traumatized site with noncrushing vascular clamps followed by close intimal approximation without lumen compromise, using interrupted vascular suture. Documentation via repeated palpation or Doppler monitoring of distal arterial flow after repair is imperative. In addition, excessive blunt intraoperative arterial trauma potentially can result in arterial spasm or intimal damage and subsequent thrombosis and arterial occlusion. Postoperative declaration of this process is dramatic, with intractable pain and discoloration of the involved extremity. Prompt removal of the propagated thrombus is mandatory and facilitated by using a balloon catheter, gaining access through a femoral incision.

Intestinal tract

Postoperative ileus is best considered a temporary annoyance for the patient rather than a significant complication of the procedure. Although nearly all patients experience some degree of ileus, prolongation probably reflects excessive manipulation and packing of the lower intestines intraoperatively and is more common and exaggerated in previously irradiated patients. Nasogastric intubation and suction are not routinely used after radical hysterectomy but are instituted when evidence of impending prolonged ileus is elicited. At that time, our choice of treatment is direction of a long (Tucker) decompression tube through the pylorus under radiologic guidance.

Occasional segmental adynamic ileus is difficult to distinguish clinically and radiologically from mechanical bowel obstruction. After long-tube decompression and a short period of intestinal inactivity, mechanical bowel obstruction is apparent and generally requires surgical correction. Intestinal obstruction after radical hysterectomy is uncommon, but it is invariably of small bowel origin; it occurs with a frequency of less than 1 % at our institution [9]. Although postoperative adhesion formation or partial volvulus are the most common causes of obstruction found at reoperation, the authors have also witnessed the herniation of small bowel into the retroperitoneum (facilitated by suction catheters in this space) through defects along the line of pelvic reperitonealization.

Intestinal fistulae are exceedingly rare and invariably occur as a recto- or sigmoidovaginal fistula in patients who have had previous irradiation. Management begins with the documentation of the intestinal source to eliminate an unrecognized small bowel communication prior to creation of a diverting colostomy in these previously irradiated patients. Reevaluation of the defect and the integrity of the adjacent tissue 3–6 months after diagnosis determines repairability and the techniques necessary to reestablish bowel continuity.

Urinary tract

Trauma and vascular compromise of the distal half of the pelvic ureter during its dissection and mobilization from the vesicouterine web will, on occasion, become clinically evident as a ureteric fistula. Although the pioneers of this procedure recognized the impact of this postoperative complication, a progressive decrease in the ureteric fistula rate has been noted, with most institutions, including Mayo [9], reporting rates approximating 1 % in nonirradiated patients. Several factors are worthy of emphasis in the prevention of ureteral fistula formation: (1) delay mobilization of ureter from the peritoneum and the vesicouterine web until near the end of the procedure, (2) use sharp dissection for mobilizing ureters from the vesicouterine web, (3) minimize trauma to the ureteral sheath containing its longitudinal blood supply, (4) minimize ureteral traction – vein retractors or natural tissue cradles are preferable when retraction is necessary – and (5) manage retroperitoneum, including vaginal vault closure and suction drainage, to minimize infection and hematoma formation. Conservative management of ureteral fistulas while waiting (3 months) for resolution of periureteral and pelvic induration and inflammation is suggested but only occasionally successful. Definitive surgical repair generally entails a tension-free ureteroneocystostomy, either alone or in the presence of a vesical psoas hitch for restoration of urinary tract continuity as described by Podratz *et al.* [16]. The ureteric fistula rate in the Mayo series was nearly five-fold higher in patients previously irradiated and was, at least in part, a reflection of the endarteritic obliteration of small vessels and fibrotic changes of the adjacent soft tissues [9]. These postirradiated periureteral changes frequently require more diverse options for surgical management, including ureteral substitutions, transureteroureterostomy, and transposition of vascular-rich tissue to secure appropriate healing.

Vesical fistulas infrequently accompany radical extirpation of the uterus unless the pelvis was previously irradiated. Sharp dissection and mobilization of the bladder base from the anterior surface of the vagina, primary vaginal closure, continuous aspiration of retroperitoneal serosanguineous fluid, and more extended postoperative gravitational drainage of the bladder presumably have contributed to these favorable results [15]. However, the vesical fistula rates in previously irradiated patients subjected to radical and 'extended' radical hysterectomies were 5 and 13%, respectively, in our series [9]. Such vesical defects result from necrosis of the surgically induced ischemia of the vulnerable bladder base and require delays of at least 3 months prior to attempts at repair. Fistula size and location as well as adjacent tissue texture dictate the approach to management. The surgeon should be familiar with various neovascularization procedures, intestinal patches, and bladder substitutions as well as suprapubic diversion techniques recently reviewed by Boronow [17].

The radicality of resection of the lateral pelvic web, vesicouterine web, and uterosacral ligaments and the extent of vaginectomy determine the type(s) and extent of bladder dysfunction after radical hysterectomy. The majority of our patients experience some degree of decreased bladder sensation, reflecting the interruption of the autonomic afferent nerves. There is also the potential for chronic bladder overdistention and secondary atony. To avoid such sequelae, all patients are encouraged to increase their micturition frequency at scheduled time intervals until adequate regenerational or substitutional mechanisms (i.e., peritoneal distention or pressure on adjacent organs) are readily and reliably recognized as signals of bladder filling. The superimposition of significant autonomic efferent denervation of the distal urinary tract can result in dysfunctional detrusor activity and the inability of the patient to empty the bladder. Again, avoiding overdistention of the bladder postoperatively is essential and it is minimized by extended gravitational drainage. Various degrees of improvement are generally observed during the subsequent 6–12 months. We prefer the incorporation of a suprapubic cystostomy at the time of operation to facilitate self-maintenance if long-term usage becomes necessary. Nevertheless, an occasional patient requires appropriate instructions in the Valsalva maneuver, with straining of accessory muscles or suprapubic Credé's method and, rarely, intermittent self-catheterization to avoid persistently increased postvoid residual urine volumes.

Postoperative urinary incontinence is more frequently associated with an intact collecting system than fistula formation. Kadar and Nelson [18] recently addressed this condition and suggested detailed radiologic and urodynamic evaluations prior to surgical repair, attempting to identify those patients demonstrating hypertonic pressures in response to bladder filling. This group is generally recalcitrant to retropubic urethropexy and warrants trials of anticholinergic agents. Our experience indicates that incontinence usually results from rotational urethral descent or a decreased continent zone secondary to excessive bladder-neck funneling after radical hysterectomies. We have used, with acceptable success, the Marshall-Marchetti-Krantz procedure for correction of hypermobility of the proximal urethra and supplemented this procedure with bladder-neck plication in those cases with excessive bladder-neck funneling. Based on earlier experiences at this institution, the authors urge delay of all surgical procedures for correction of incontinence not related to fistula formation for at least 1 year after the original radical operative procedure.

Evaluation of treatment

The indications for radical hysterectomy and pelvic lymphadenectomy at our institution have not changed appreciably over the past three decades and, with rare exception, the procedure has been used as primary therapy in patients who have clinical stage IB 'occult', IB, and IIA cervical carcinoma. This surgical approach was initially forwarded with the conviction that radical extirpation is at least as efficacious as radiotherapy and also allows preservation of ovarian function, more accurate assessment of disease, avoidance of long-term bowel and bladder sequelae, and deferment of an effective modality (radiotherapy) for treatment of recurrent disease. These advantages continue to be recognized by contemporary pelvic surgeons. Presumably reflecting subtle changes in epidemiologic factors, we have witnessed a progressive decrease in the median age at which cervical carcinoma has become clinically evident; therefore, the necessity for conserving ovaries is even more relevant today. Likewise, the merits of definitive 'surgical staging' are acknowledged and more recently also incorporated with regularity in the pretreatment evaluation of patients with more advanced disease. In addition, the often cited major disadvantages of the surgical approach, namely, the higher mortality and morbidity rates, are of lesser impact today than several decades ago. Continued technologic and medical advances, particularly in postoperative monitoring, nutritional support, and microbial control, have resulted in continued improvement in treatment-related mortality, as exemplified by the 0.3% 30-day operative mortality (610 patients) at our institution between 1956 and 1975 [9]. Advances and alterations in surgical technique (including primary vaginal closure and closed-catheter drainage) [15] have dramatically decreased major surgical morbidity and hospitalization time. Furthermore, the major surgical complications that occasionally surface after radical hysterectomy are generally amenable to appropriate correction.

Patient survival 5 years after completion of treatment routinely serves as an indicator of therapeutic effectiveness and is generally reported according to the clinical stage of the disease. The longevity of the Mayo population based on 5-year survival rates was: stage IA, 96%; IB, 90%; IIA, 69%; and IIB, 52% [9]. Although these results compare favorably with those from other institutions, the authors think there is only marginal value in attempting to evaluate surgical (or other) treatment of early cervical carcinoma according to clinical stage. Any staging process should entail the precise indexing of the extent of neoplastic involvement, accurately reflect the natural history of the disease, and form the basis for individual therapy, prognosis, and comparative evaluation. The current FIGO clinical staging does not discriminate occult involvement of the parametrium, embolization to pelvic lymph nodes, or extrapelvic metastases frequently detected at surgical exploration and staging. For example, nodal involvement was observed in 14% of clinical stage IB and 27% of stage IIA patients at our institution, with corresponding 5-year survival rates of 57% in those patients who had positive nodes compared with 83% when nodes were negative [9]. Martimbeau *et al.* [19] subsequently noted similar survival rates (53 and 92%, respectively) according to nodal involvement in patients (562) with clinical stage IB disease and they observed a significant difference in survivorship when common iliac nodes were positive (14%) as opposed to external iliac nodes (65%). Furthermore, Bleker *et al.* [20] reported a progressive decrease in 5-year survival rates in patients with stages IB and IIA cervical carcinoma having local disease only (90%), parametrial extension only (75%), nodal embolization only (62%), and both parametrial and nodal involvement (50%). No differences in survival rates were noted between patients with clinical stages IB and IIA if surgical or pathologic evaluation demonstrated disease beyond the confines of the endopelvic fascia. Although interinstitutional comparative evaluations of treatment modalities by using clinical staging in large series of early cervical carcinoma find continued acceptance, the assessment of the influence of specific histologic parameters and evaluation of primary therapeutic effectiveness as well as selection of adjuvant therapy require accurate surgical staging if patients at risk are to realize improved survivorship.

When treatment-associated morbidity is deemed acceptable, the most reliable indicator of the effectiveness of a chosen therapeutic modality and the expertise with which it is administered is the rate of recurrence of the disease. In the Mayo series of 564 patients with cervical carcinoma who were subjected to radical hysterectomy and pelvic lymphadenectomy, including 141 previously irradiated patients with persistent disease, the overall recurrence rate was 18% [21]. Although pelvic sidewall and distant recurrences presumably reflect suboptimal diagnostic capabilities, primary pelvic lymphadenectomy or postoperative adjuvant therapy, and tumor biology, the most cogent factor in evaluating the effectiveness of the radical hysterectomy is the frequency of central pelvic recurrences. Assessment of the initial sites of failure in our population demonstrated 49 patients with pelvic recurrences only (8.7%), 12 with pelvic and extrapelvic sites (2.1%), and 43 with extrapelvic failures only (7.6%). Further analysis showed only 20 patients (3.5%) had recurrent disease involving the central pelvis and in only nine of these patients (1.6%) was the failure isolated to the central pelvis only.

Whereas only 9% of patients with recurrent carcinoma demonstrated isolated central pelvic disease, 38% had pelvic sidewall recurrence (with or without central disease) and 53% had recurrent disease outside the pelvis [21]. The most important surgical or pathologic factor for predicting regional and distant failures was nodal metastases at the time of primary lymphadenectomy; 35% of patients with pelvic sidewall recurrences and 43% with extrapelvic recurrences had pelvic nodal involvement originally. Furthermore, 40% of patients with primary nodal disease who had radical hysterectomy and pelvic node dissection eventually were declared treatment failures, suggesting potential value in postoperative adjuvant therapy in this identifiable group. However, the role of postoperative whole pelvic irradiation in this high-risk population has been explored at several institutions [19, 22, 23], with no significant decrease in the overall survival rate. Review of the sites of failure of the Mayo population [21] predicts a maximum of only 15% of the patients with positive pelvic nodes who would potentially have been afforded additional curative benefits when supplemented with irradiation and only a fraction of the 25% who had extrapelvic recurrences might have anticipated some enhancement in regional control. Therefore, with the apparent propensity of patients with nodal involvement to harbor occult disseminated disease, the incorporation of systemic chemotherapy in the overall treatment of this subset of patients appears rational, with preliminary results of using cisplatin and bleomycin justifying phase III clinical trials [24].

The frequency of treatment failure in patients who had radical hysterectomy and negative pelvic lymphadenectomy was 14% at our institution [21]. Sites of recurrences were nearly equally distributed between the pelvis alone and extrapelvic locations (with or without simultaneous pelvic recurrences). Again, the selective use of postoperative adjuvant therapy appears reasonable but will require identification of a high-risk subset with sufficient sensitivity and specificity to minimize unnecessary exposure to additional therapy. In the absence of nodal involvement, other surgical or pathologic characteristics including lesion size [25–28], parametrial involvement [20], depth of stromal invasion [29], histologic and cellular subtypes [26, 28, 30, 31], and capillary-like space involvement [28, 32, 33] have been associated with less favorable prognoses and may be used singly or as a battery in identifying patients at significant risk for developing recurrent disease who are, therefore, candidates for additional therapy.

The postrecurrent 5-year salvage rate of 6% in our patient population [21] demonstrates the absolute necessity for comprehensive primary therapy, including effective postoperative adjuvant therapy in patients at high risk for recurrent disease. However, the various adjuvant therapeutic modalities, used independently or in combination, must withstand the intense scrutiny of appropriately controlled clinical trials prior to general implementation, including analysis of the sensitivity and specificity of patient selection to minimize additional unwarranted morbidity.

References

1. Wertheim E. 1912. The extended abdominal operation for carcinoma uteri (based on 500 operative cases). Am J Obstet (NY) 66:169–232.
2. Meigs JV. 1944. Carcinoma of the cervix – the Wertheim operation. Surg Gynecol Obstet 78:195–199.
3. Meigs JV. 1951. Radical hysterectomy with bilateral pelvic lymph node dissections. A report of 100 patients operated on five or more years ago. Am J Obstet Gynecol 62:854–865.
4. Roddick JW Jr, Greenelaw RH. 1971. Treatment of cervical cancer: a randomized study of operation and radiation. Am J Obstet Gynecol 109:754–759.
5. Newton M. 1975. Radical hysterectomy or radiotherapy for stage I cervical cancer: a prospective comparison with 5 and 10 year follow-up. Am J Obstet Gynecol 123:535–539.
6. Morley GW, Seski JC. 1976. Radical pelvic surgery versus radiation therapy for stage I carcinoma of the cervix (exclusive of microinvasion). Am J Obstet Gynecol 126:785–794.

7. van Nagell JR Jr, Roddick JW Jr, Lowin DM. 1971. The staging of cervical cancer: inevitable discrepancies between clinical staging and pathologic findings. Am J Obstet Gynecol 110:973–978.
8. Symmonds RE, Pratt JH, Welch JS. 1964. Extended Wertheim operation for primary, recurrent, or suspected recurrent carcinoma of the cervix. Obstet Gynecol 24:15–24.
9. Webb MJ, Symmonds RE. 1979. Wertheim hysterectomy: a reappraisal. Obstet Gynecol 54:140–145.
10. Cavanagh D, Rutledge F. 1960. The cervical cone biopsy-hysterectomy sequence and factors affecting the febrile morbidity. Am J Obstet Gynecol 80:53–59.
11. Malinak LR, Jeffrey RA Jr, Dunn WJ. 1964. The conization-hysterectomy time interval: a clinical and pathologic study. Obstet Gynecol 23:317–329.
12. Mikuta JJ, Giuntoli RL, Rubin EL, Mangan CE. 1977. The 'problem' radical hysterectomy. Am J Obstet Gynecol 128:119–124.
13. Webb MJ, Symmonds RE. 1979. Radical hysterectomy: influence of recent conization on morbidity and complications. Obstet Gynecol 53:290–292.
14. McIlrath DC, van Heerden JA, Edis AJ, Dozois RR. 1976. Closure of abdominal incisions with subcutaneous catheters. Surgery 80:411–415.
15. Symmonds RE, Pratt JH. 1961. Prevention of fistulas and lymphocysts in radical hysterectomy: preliminary report of a new technic. Obstet Gynecol 17:57–64.
16. Podratz KC, Angerman NS, Symmonds RE. 1982. Complications of ureteral surgery in the nonradiated patient. In: Management of Complications in Gynecologic Oncology. Edited by G Delgado, JP Smith. New York, John Wiley & Sons, pp 113–149.
17. Boronow RC. 1982. Urologic complications secondary to radiation alone or radiation and surgery. In: Management of Complications in Gynecologic Oncology (G Delgado, JP Smith, eds). John Wiley & Sons, New York, pp 163-197.
18. Kadar N, Nelson JH Jr. 1984. Treatment of urinary incontinence after radical hysterectomy. Obstet Gynecol 64:400–405.
19. Martimbeau PW, Kjorstad KE, Iversen T. 1982. Stage IB carcinoma of the cervix, The Norwegian Radium Hospital. II. Results when pelvic nodes are involved. Obstet Gynecol 60:215–218.
20. Bleker OP, Ketting BW, van Wayjen-Eecen B, Kloosterman GJ. 1983. The significance of microscopic involvement of the parametrium and/or pelvic lymph nodes in cervical cancer Stages IB and IIA. Gynecol Oncol 16:56–62.
21. Webb MJ, Symmonds RE. 1980. Site of recurrence of cervical cancer after radical hysterectomy. Am J Obstet Gynecol 138:813–817.
22. Niloff JM, Bast RC Jr, Schaetzl EM, Knapp RC. 1985. Predictive value of CA 125 antigen levels in second-look procedures for ovarian cancer. Am J Obstet Gynecol 151:981–985.
23. Fuller AF Jr, Elliott N, Kosloff C, Lewis JL Jr. 1982. Lymph node metastases from carcinoma of the cervix, Stages IB and IIA: implications for prognosis and treatment. Gynecol Oncol 13:165–174.
24. Wertheim MS, Hakes TB, Daghestani AN, Nori D, Smith DH, Lewis JL Jr. 1985. A pilot study of adjuvant therapy in patients with cervical cancer at high risk of recurrence after radical hysterectomy and pelvic lymphadenectomy. J Clin Oncol 3:912–916.
25. Piver MS, Chung WS. 1975. Prognostic significance of cervical lesion size and pelvic node metastases in cervical carcinoma. Obstet Gynecol 46:507–510.
26. van Nagell JR Jr, Donaldson ES, Parker JC, van Dyke AH, Wood EG. 1977. The prognostic significance of cell type and lesion size in patients with cervical cancer treated by radical surgery. Gynecol Oncol 5:142–151.
27. Burghardt E, Pickel H. 1978. Local spread and lymph node involvement in cervical cancer. Obstet Gynecol 52:138–145.
28. van Nagell JR Jr, Rayburn W, Donaldson ES, Hanson M, Gay EC, Yoneda J, Marayuma Y, Powell DF. 1979. Therapeutic implications of patterns of recurrence in cancer of the uterine cervix. Cancer 44:2354–2361.

29. Boyce J, Fruchter RG, Nicastri AD, Ambiavagar P-C, Reinis MS, Nelson JH Jr. 1981. Prognostic factors in Stage I carcinoma of the cervix. Gynecol Oncol 12:154–165.
30. Gallup DG, Abell MR. 1977. Invasive adenocarcinoma of the uterine cervix. Obstet Gynecol 49:596–603.
31. Tamimi HK, Figge DC. 1982. Adenocarcinoma of the uterine cervix. Gynecol Oncol 13:335–344.
32. van Nagell JR Jr, Donaldson ES, Wood EG, Parker JC Jr. 1978. The significance of vascular invasion and lymphocytic infiltration in invasive cervical cancer. Cancer 41:228–234.
33. Barber HRK, Sommers SC, Rotterdam H, Kwon T. 1978. Vascular invasion as a prognostic factor in Stage IB cancer of the cervix. Obstet Gynecol 52:343–348.

7. Treatment of locally advanced cancer of the cervix with interstitial parametrial implants

SILVIO A. ARISTIZABAL

Introduction

Radiation therapy constitutes the main treatment modality in patients with locally advanced carcinoma of the cervix. Despite significant advances in equipment and techniques during the last three decades, and a better understanding of tumor radiobiology, the results remain unsatisfactory. Failure to control the primary tumor is still the most common cause of death in these women.

Efforts to improve the curability by delivering higher doses of external and/or intracavitary radiation, using conventional techniques have been disappointing. This has usually resulted in a significant increase in morbidity with no parallel improvement in tumor control rates.

The brachytherapy component of a course of treatment is the critical factor in controlling central pelvic disease because it has the radiobiological advantage of continuous low dose rate irradiation coupled with a high dose to the cervix and paracervical areas with a rapidly diminishing dose to the bladder and rectum. It would therefore seem logical, to focus attention on increasing the efficiency of the brachytherapy part of the treatment plan.

The pear-shaped dose distribution obtained with conventional intracavitary applicators (tandem and ovoid) generally adequately encompasses the tumor volume in the early stages of disease. However, the geometry of advanced tumors adversely influences tumor kill at the periphery of disease because of the abrupt reduction in dose rate with small increases in distance with these applicators. In addition, distorted anatomy, commonly associated with advanced tumors, interferes with optimum distribution of the radiation sources when using standard intracavitary applicators.

These limitations have been long recognized and attempts at improving local tumor control through modifications of the brachytherapy technique are well documented in the literature. Several investigators have reported improved results in advanced carcinoma of the cervix by direct implanta-

E.A. Surwit, D.S. Alberts (eds) Cervix Cancer.

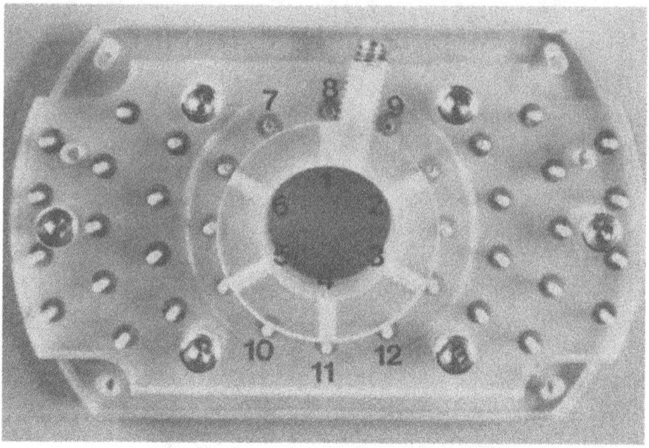

Figure 1. Perineal template. Positions of needles on the surface of the vaginal cylinder are numbers 1–6. Positions number 7–9 and 10–12 are bladder and rectal needles, respectively.

tion of 'hot' radium needles into the cervix and parametrium to supplement the dose to those areas [4–7]. Unfortunately, radiation protection hazards and dosimetric difficulties with radium needles make this approach impractical and unacceptable. More recently, the availability of new isotopes with significant radiation protection advantages and the introduction of afterloading techniques have greatly improved radiation safety. This, combined with the expedience of accuracy of computerized dosimetry has contributed for renewed interest in interstitial brachytherapy.

A new procedure which incorporates all these new technical developments [8], has been used at our institution for the treatment of locally advanced cancer of the cervix for the past 7 years.

The transperineal implant

The procedure employs a plastic template with pre-drilled holes in concentric rows at one centimeter intervals. A larger central opening in the template accepts a plastic cylinder 2 cm in diameter, 15 cm long (vaginal candle), which has a central opening for the placement of a conventional uterine tandem. There are 38 holes in the template, and an additional six needles fit into grooves on the periphery of the vaginal cylinder. A 4 cm × 10 cm area can be implanted with this needle configuration in combination, if desired, with placement of a vaginal-uterine tandem (Figure 1).

The procedure is always done under general or spinal anesthesia with the patient in the dorso lithotomy position; it requires a careful perineal and vaginal preparation. A foley cathether is passed into the bladder and the

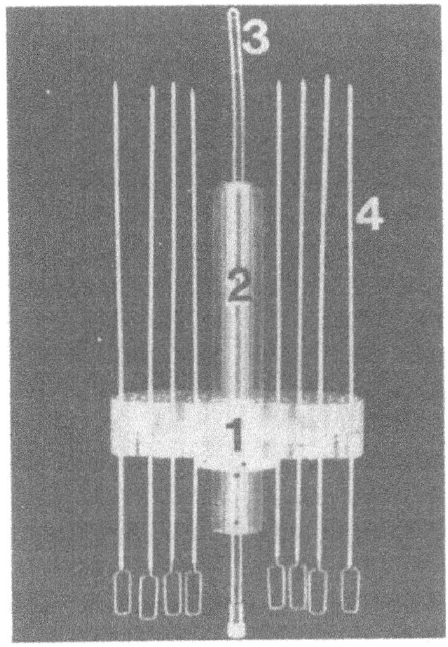

Figure 2. Peineal template (1), vatinal cylinder (2), uterine tandem (3), and interstitial needles (4) assembly, showing how the template keeps the needles parallel to each other and fixed at the chosen depth.

balloon is filled with radioopaque fluid. Recto-vaginal examination is mandatory prior to the procedure, to assess the tumor shape and volume, to facilitate the positioning of the first needle, and to check the depth of insertion. A uterine tandem is inserted in the same fashion as in standared intracavitary application. The vaginal cylinder is threaded over the tandem and advanced until it comes in contact with the external cervical os. Now the template is slipped over the cylinder and placed against the perineal surface. The different components are fixed into position by tightening machine screws. The 17-gauge, 20 cm long, hollow metal or plastic needles, are inserted through the holes in the template across the perineum and advanced into the para-cervical areas to a preselected depth beyong the cervix, which depends on the bulkiness of the tumor (Figure 2). When inserting the most central posterior needles, frequent rectal examination are important to rule-out rectal penetration. If rectal entry is demonstrated, the relevant needle is repositioned or removed permanently. If a tandem is not used, then a concentric row of needles is placed in the six grooves on the surface of the vaginal obturator (Figure 1, positions 1–6). Tightening of four machine screws fix all the needles to the template, at the chosen depth.

Orthogonal verification films (Figure 3), are taken in the Radiation Oncology Department with dummy sources in the guide needles. The patient is

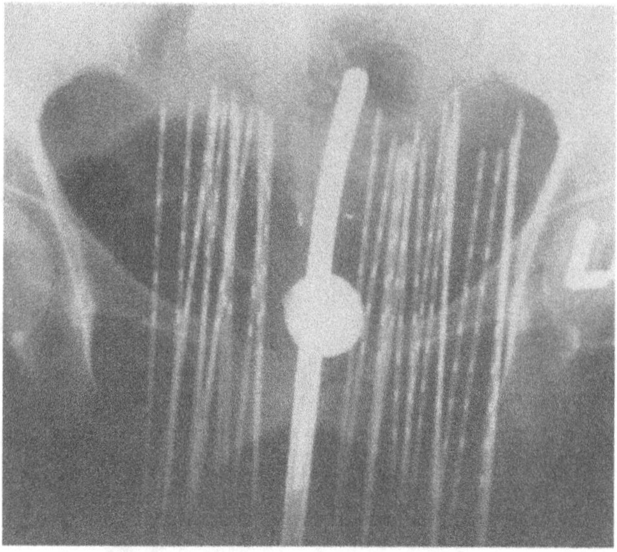

Figure 3. Anteroposterior and lateral orthogonal radiographs for a stage IIIB patient with residual tumor in the left lateral parametrium and left uterosacral ligament, at the time of the implant. Patient is alive and without evidence of disease 6 years post-treatment.

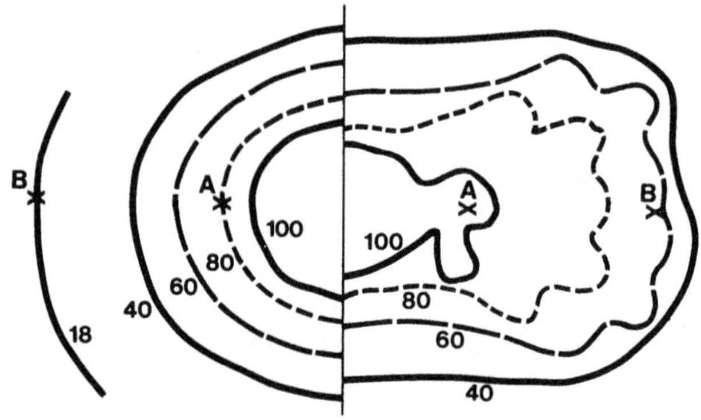

Figure 4. A transverse cut of computerized isodose distributions for tandem and ovoids (T and Os) and interstitial implant, at the level of points A and B.

then returned to her room for afterloading of the radioactive sources. The intrauterine tandem is loaded in the standard way with 226-Radium or 137-Cesium capsules. 192-Iridium or 137-Cesium microsources are loaded into the implanted needles. If there is no bulky residual tumor or disease in the anterior and/or posterior fornices the rectal and bladder needles are not loaded (Figure 1, positions 7–9 and 10–12). Three-dimensional computer dosimetry is used to generate isodose plots around the implanted volume and to calculate doses to any point of interest within the pelvis (Figure 4).

Once irradiation is completed and the radioactive sources have been removed, the whole implant (template, needle guides, vaginal cylinder and tandem) can be removed in one motion with little difficulty. Light sedation is usually adequate.

Dosimetric considerations

At the University of Arizona, most patients had an intrauterine tandem inserted and loaded in conjunction with the implant. Eventhough loading of the tandem produces a 'hot spot' in the center of the implant, this inhomogeneity is advantageous if we take into consideration: (1) the higher radiation tolerance of the uterus and cervix; (2) the frequent presence of residual tumor in this central location at the time of the brachytherapy procedure; (3) the possibility, in some patients, of tumor extension into the lower uterine segment and/or endometrial cavity; and (4) the dose contribution from the tandem to the regional pelvic nodes. Moreover, reported results from the University of Maryland suggested a more favorable outcome in patients who had a tandem loaded in conjunction with the parametrial implant [7]. Finally, an additional advantage of having a tandem in place, is that it provides good stabilization and alignment for the vaginal cylinder and template.

Comparison of localization radiographs and isodose distributions from conventional tandem and ovoids versus interstitial implants have demonstrated significant differences between the two systems (Figure 4). For example, the template system irradiates a greater length of the rectal wall, and hence, tolerance levels are not necessarily synonimous with the two systems. Since clinical experience with the interstitial implant was limited and dosimetric guidelines nonexistant it was elected, to record doses to points A and B, and also, milligram hour values in addition to the three-dimensional isodose curves.

Methods and materials

From July 1978 to June 1981, an initial pilot study, using the transperineal approach as described by Feder and Syed [8], was done at the University of Arizona (UA). A detailed account of the patients treated has been previously published [9]. The preliminary results confirmed improvement in pelvic control rates in both stage IIB and IIIB patients. The improved results however, had been obtained at the expense of a marked increase in severe complications. Consequently, the second phase of the study was carefully designed to introduce gradual changes in technique and dosimetry in an effort to reduce the morbidity while preserving the improvement in local control.

Between July 1981 and June 1982, during the author's sabattical year, a prospective investigation was carried out at the University of El Valle (UV) in Cali-Colombia [10]. One hundred patients with carcinoma of the cervix stage IIB and IIIB were treated in a systematic way. Technical and dosimetric modifications were introduced one at a time and only when warranted by previous clinical observations. To minimize the number of treatment variables, all patients were given similar doses of external irradiation (Cobalt-60 unit, 80 cm SSD; 167 rad per fraction $\times$ 30 to 5000 rad; TDF: 75), to the whole pelvis plus a parametrial boost of 500 rad in 3 fractions, for a total of 5500 rad. The interstitial volume was kept constant by implanting the whole width of the pelvis in every patient, irrespective of tumor size and stage, and by using 137-Cesium reusable microsources with a fixed active length of 6 cm. The tandem was loaded in a standard way with 30 to 35 mgr Radium equivalent (mRe), 137-Cesium capsules. Only one implant procedure was done per patient.

The average number of needles inserted per patients was 30. Since the activity of the 137-Cesium microsources was 2.2 mRe, the average amount of activity in all the implanted needles was 66 mRe. A close correlation was noted between the total mRe in the implant (including the 30–35 mRe in the tandem), and the dose rate to point A (90 to 100 rad per hour). The corresponding dose rate at homolateral point B was 50 to 60% of that at point A (Figure 4). The implant was left in place for 48 hrs or 4800 mg hrs; the average dose to point A was 4800 rad and to point B, between 2400 and 2800 rad.

Of the 26 patients treated at the UA, six underwent concurrent laparotomy with the implant procedure. In addition, 18 patients underwent either one intracavitary application and one interstitial implant, or two interstitial procedures, performed two weeks apart. Furthermore, in most UA patients, 192-Iridium seeds in plastic-tubing carriers were used. The Iridium ribbons have an advantage over the Cesium sources in that they can be custom ordered or cut at 1 cm increments, to obtain the desired active length for a specific need.

Individualized treatment, an important factor in optimization of results, was not available to the 98 patients who received radiotherapy at the UV. Because of heavy machine usage during external radiation, only one field was treated every day; only one implant procedure was planned per patient; reusable, 137-Cesium microsources, 6 cm fixed active length, were substituted for the Iridium ribbons. In contrast, at the UA, every field was treated each day; most patients with gross residual tumor at the time of the interstitial implant received two brachytherapy procedures.

The majority of the patients were evaluated prior to treatment and followed at 6-month intervals by the author (S.A.). Mean follow-up for the entire group is 36 months. Four patients, one stage IIB and three stage IIIB, have been lost to follow-up less than 1 year from completion of treatment.

Results in stage IIB

Only patients who had parametrial involvement without fixation to the pelvic wall are classified as IIB (FIGO). Patients with lesions expanding the lower uterine segment to a size equal or greater than 6 cm, so-called 'barrel' tumors, were included only if extension into the parametrial areas was present at diagnosis. Large, everting exophytic masses, 6 cm or greater, without lower uterine segment involvement, were labeled 'bulky' lesions.

Primary control of pelvic disease was accomplished in 82% (37/45) of the patients. Table 1 summarizes local failure rates as a function of several prognostic factors. Local recurrence rates, either centrally or in the parametrial and pelvic wall areas, were similar in patients with bulky tumors or lesions less than 6 cm in size (10% and 13% respectively). Patients with 'barrel' shaped tumors, however, had a high rate of local failure (3/5 or 60%).

Pelvic failure rates appeared to be inversely related to the extent of parametrium involvement; patients with medial parametrium extension showed

Table 1. Prognostic factors versus local failure in stage II B.

Factor	No. of patients	Local failure	Significance level (p-value)
Tumor size			
<6 cm	30	4/30 (13%)	
≥6 cm	15	4/15 (26%)	0.270
'Bulky'	10	1/10 (10%)	
'Barrel'	5	3/5 (60%)	0.03
Parametrium involvement			
Medial*	15	2/15 (13%)	
Distal	23	3/23 (13%)	0.315
Age (years)			
≤45	22	6/22 (27.0%)	
>45	23	2/23 (6.7%)	0.103
Histology			
Squamous cell	38	7/38 (18.4%)	
Adenocarcinoma	6	1/16 (16.6%)	0.918

* Patients with 'barrel shaped' tumors, excluded.

a 25% local recurrence rate, while in those with involvement of the lateral parametrium the failure rate was only 13%. The discrepancy however, disappeared when patients with 'barrel' tumors were excluded from analysis; the local recurrence rates became quite similar for the two groups (2/15 or 13% and 3/23 or 13%).

The influence of patient age on local failure in our series was confounded by its relationship to tumor size, since all 'barrel' tumors and 2/3 of the 'bulky' lesions occurred in patients 45 years of age or younger. Twenty seven percent of these patients recurred locally compared with 6.7% recurrence rate in patients older than 45 years of age.

No correlation was found between pelvic failure rate and histology of tumor. Local recurrence rates were essentially the same for squamous cell and adenocarcinomas, 18.4 and 16.6% respectively.

The prognostic value of tumor response recorded at the time of te first brachytherapy application was also investigated and the results are illustrated in Table 2. There were no local failures in patients who had a complete tumor response prior to the implant procedure while 26% (8/31) of patients with gross residual tumor at the time of the interstitial implant, failed locally ($p = 0.002$). Moreover, when local recurrence rate was examined as a function of the number of brachytherapy procedures, no recurrences were found in a subset of patients with gross residual tumor, who underwent two brachytherapy procedures (0/6), versus 32% (8/25) failures in similar patients who had only one interstitial implant. The small number of patients may have prevented this difference from achieving statistical significance ($p = 0.108$).

Results in stage IIIB

Only patients with tumor extension and fixation to the pelvic wall were included under this category. Patients classified as stage IIIB because of hydronephrosis (FIGO), but without fixation to the pelvic wall, were excluded from this analysis. Tumors with a large, central exophytic component, 6 cm or greater were subgrouped as 'bulky' lesions.

Table 2. Tumor response versus local failure in stage II B.

Response	No. of patients		No. branchytherapy procedures	Local failure	Significance level (p-value)
Complete	14		1	0/14 (0%)	
Partial	31			8/31 (26%)	0.020
		25	1	8/25 (32%)	
		6	2	0/6 (0%)	0.108

The correlation of pelvic failure with various prognostic factors in stage IIIB patients is listed in Table 3. The size of the central tumor had no influence in the local control rates; patients with 'bulky' disease recurred at the same rate as those classified as 'non-bulky' (26% and 23% respectively). On the other hand, peripheral tumor extension to both pelvic walls and/or distal vagina seemed to worsen the prognosis. The local recurrence increased from 17% in patients with no vaginal involvement, to 30% in those with tumor extending into the distal vagina. Likewise, the 20% pelvic failure rate observed in patients with unilateral pelvic wall fixation rose to 33% in those with bilateral fixation.

The presence of hydronephrosis also adversely affected the results. The local failure rate in patients with normal excretory urograms was 22% while 30% and 75% of patients with unilateral and bilateral hydronephrosis, respectively, developed local recurrence ($p = 0.028$).

The influence of patients age on the pelvic outcome was also studied. Patients younger than 45 years of age appeared to have a significantly worse

Table 3. Prognostic factors versus local failure in stage III B.

Factor	No. of patients	Local failure	Significance level (p-value)
Tumor size			
Non bulky	57	13/57 (23.0%)	
Bulky	27	7/27 (26.0%)	0.754
Pelvic-wall fixation			
Unilateral	63	13/63 (20.6%)	
Bilateral	21	7/21 (33.0%)	0.237
Vaginal involvement			
No	23	4/23 (17.4%)	
Yes	61	16/61 (26.0%)	0.396
Distal 1/3	10	3/10 (30.0%)	0.416
Hydronephrosis			
No	64	14/64 (22.0%)	
Yes	20	6/20 (30.0%)	0.456
Unilateral	16	3/16 (18.7%)	
Bilateral	4	3/4 (75.0%)	0.028
No vs. unilateral vs. bilateral			0.047
Age			
<45	31	11/31 (35.5%)	
>45	53	9/53 (17.0%)	0.055
Histology			
Squamous-cell	79	20/79 (26.6%)	
Adenocarcinoma	5	0/5 (00.0%)	0.197

prognosis, with a rate of local recurrence twice as high (35.5%) as that of the older patients (17%, $p = 0.055$).

To investigate the impact of tumor response to external radiation on the pelvic failure rate, patients were subgrouped according to pelvic findings at the time of the interstitial implant procedure (Table 4). Patients with minimal or no evidence of residual tumor were classified as having a complete response (CR). Those with gross residual tumor were classified either as partial responders (PR), when there had been at least a 50% reduction in the size of the palpable and visible lesion, or non responders (NR), when only minimal or no changes, had occurred in the size of original tumor. A statistically significant difference in the recurrence rate of these subgroups of patients was observed. The local recurrence rate increased from 0% to 21.7% to 58% in patients with CR, PR and NR respectively ($p = 0.039$). The number of brachy-therapy procedures appeared to influence the rate of local failure in patients with residual disease (24% and 15% with one and two interstitial implants, respectively); eventhough the results are not statistically significant they nevertheless suggest that, patients with gross residual tumor may benefit from two procedures.

No significant correlation was found between the histology of the tumor (squamous-cell vs. adenocarcinoma) and local recurrence rates.

Complications

Complications were classified according to the following guidelines:

grade I: mild transient symptoms of enteritis, proctosigmoiditis, cystitis, etc. that responded to conservative medical treatment;

grade II: severe and/or persistent episodes of proctosigmoiditis, enteritis, cystitis; recurrent hemthochezia or hematuria; vaginal ulcer, localized necrosis. Symptoms improved with conservative medical treatment;

grade III: fistulization and other complications requiring surgical intervention;

Table 4. Tumor response versus local failure in stage III B.

Response	No. of patients	No. brachytherapy procedures	Local failure	Significance level (p-value)
CR	11	1 or 2	0/11 (00.0%)	
PR	46		10/46 (21.7%)	
	33	1	8/33 (24.0%)	
	13	2	2/13 (15.0%)	0.512
NR	12	1 or 2	7/12 (58.0%)	

CR = complete response; PR = partial response; NR = no response.
CR vs. PR vs. NR, $p = 0.004$; CR vs. PR/NR, $p = 0.039$.

grade IV: death resulting from treatment or as a result of radiation injury to normal organs.

About one-third of the patients (30%) developed grade I side effects. Since these side effects were mild and transient in nature and medical treatment resulted in complete recovery, they were not included in further analysis of complications. Fifteen patients (11.4%), experienced grade II complications and severe side effects (grade III) were recorded in an additional 15 patients (11.4%). Thus, the frequency of serious radiation morbidity (grade II-III) was 22.8%. There were no fatal radiation related complications.

The frequency and severity of complications by institution, by clinical stage, and as a function of milligram hours and geometry of implant is shown in Table 5. Patients treated at the University of Arizona had a 32% incidence of complications, 80% of them were grade III; in contrast, the rate of complications in patients treated at the University of El Valle was 20% and only 35% were grade III type. The frequency and severity of the complications at the UA is a reflection of several factors including staging laparotomy in six patients and/or placement of radioactive sources on the surface of the vaginal obturator in conjunction with a loaded tandem in seven patients (Table 6). Eight of these eleven patients (72.7%), developed complications, most of them severe, while in the remaining patients the complication rate was significantly lower, 18.6% (22/118, $p = 0.005$).

When analyzed, by clinical stage, mg-hrs and implant geometry, no difference in the frequency and severity of complications was apparent.

Table 5. Analysis of complications.

			Grade (%)	
Factor	No. of patients	Complication rate	II	III
Institution				
Univ. of Arizona	31	10/31 (32.0%)	20.0	80.0
Univ. of El Valle	98	20/98 (20.4%)	65.0	35.0
Stage				
II B	45	10/45 (22.0%)	60.0	40.0
III B	84	20/84 (23.8%)	45.0	55.0
Total mg-hrs				
<4,500	47	8/47 (17.0%)	62.5	37.5
>4,500	82	22/82 (26.8%)	60.0	40.0
Geometry				
Standard	50	9/50 (18.0%)	66.6	33.0
Modified	48	11/48 (23.0%)	64.0	36.0
Number Inplants				
1	113	20/113 (17.7%)	60.0	40.0
2	25	9/25 (36.6%)	22.2	77.7

Table 6. Treatment factors and complications.

Factor	No. of patients	Complication rate	Significance level (p-value)
Laparotomy only	4	2/4 (50.0%)	
obturator needles only	5	4/5 (80.0%)	
Laparotomy and obturator	2	2/2 (100.0%)	
No laparotomy or obturator	118	22/118 (18.6%)	0.0005

Discussion

Stage IIB

Historically, local failure in patients with stage IIB carcinoma of the cervix treated with external megavoltage irradiation and conventional intracavitary applicators (tandem and ovoid) ranges from 15 to 30% [11–15]. The 17% pelvic recurrence rate in our series of patients treated with interstitial implants, therefore compares favorably with these reported results.

However, stage IIB cervical cancer is a wide spectrum of disease that includes patients with both medial and lateral parametrial invasion. The cervix may look normal in size or be markedly expanded to 6 cm or more. The tumor may be of the exophytic, ulcerative or endophytic type and in the latter case it may produce marked expansion and distortion of the lower uterine segment. The radiocurability of these various lesions differ, some even requiring adjunctive hysterectomy to secure local control of the disease [12, 16, 17]. It is therefore extremely important in the evaluation of the interstitial technique, to examine, not only the overall results, but also its relative efficacy in subsets of patients with differing prognoses.

Endophytic lesions arising in the endocervix with expansion of the lower uterine segment ('barrel shaped' tumor), have long been recognized as a separate entity with a very high risk for local recurrence [12, 16, 18]. Nelson and coworkers concluded that the 'barrel shaped lesion was the principal indication for combining radiotherapy and hysterectomy'. The rational was, that the hysterectomy removed the tumor in the lower uterine segment which did not receive an effective dose from the intracavitary radium system. With this combined approach central failures were almost entirely eliminated [19].

Post-radiation hysterectomy for 'barrel' lesions was not part of our parametrial implant study; as shown in Table 1, the local failure rate in our series was 60% (3/5). One possible explanation for this high recurrence rate, is that with the implant the effective irradiated volume is stretched laterally while 'barrel' lesions have the tendency to infiltrate superiorly into the uterus. Thus, our results suggest that interstitial implants are not a satisfactory substitute for hysterectomy following radiation in patients with 'barrel shaped' tumors.

Bulky exopytic tumors, with a large central component (6 cm or greater), have been found in numerous series [11, 20, 21] to be associated with a higher rate of local recurrence. Several authors have suggested an extrafascial hysterectomy after irradiation to improve local control rates [20, 21]. In our series, only 10% (1/10) of patients with bulky exophytic tumors treated with interstitial implants, have failed locally. This figure compares favorably with the 13% rate of recurrence seen in similarly treated patients, but with smaller tumors (less than 6 cm).

The rate of tumor regression to external radiation, has been found by several investigators, to be a predictor of ultimate tumor control [15, 20, 22, 23]. Furthermore, the evaluation of tumor response prior to intracavitary radiation is advantageous since, subsequent treatment may be guided in a way which will benefit the poor responders. The results in our interstitial implant patients not only confirmed the prognostic value of tumor response (0% versus 25% pelvic failure in patients with complete and partial tumor response respectively), but suggest that patients with gross residual tumor at the time of the first brachytherapy procedure would benefit from a second implant. No recurrences have been observed in patients with supoptimal tumor response who underwent two brachytherapy procedures while 32% of similar cases who had only one interstitial implant recurred locally.

Thus, evaluation of tumor response, preferably done under anesthesia in the operating room at the time of the first nrachytherapy application, is in our experience an important criteria for individualization of therapy. Patients with gross residual tumor, centrally located and who are medically operable should be considered for post-radiation hysterectomy. Similar cases who refuse surgery, are inoperable or have parametrial residual tumor should be treated with two fractionated interstitial implants, two weeks apart.

Eventhough patients age did not appear to be of prognostic value in our study a significant correlation was established: all 'barrel' lesions and 2/3 of the 'bulky' tumors (both associated with high risk of local recurrence) occurred in patients 45 years of age or younger. Similarly, in a recent review of cervical carcinoma from the University of Florida, the investigators found that patient's age was of prognostic value only when analyzed in conjunction with tumor size; younger patients had a significant higher risk of local failure [20].

Finally, neither histology or extent of parametrial involvement at diagnosis was found to be of prognostic significance in stage IIB patients in this study of patients treated with interstitial implants.

Stage IIIB

The overall pelvic failure rate in patients with stage IIIB carcinomas have remained static since the 1950's when the introduction of megavoltage radiation produced a modest improvement in results. Paunier *et al.* [25], found 218 pelvic recurrences in 599 patients (36.4%) with stage IIIB (FIGO), treated with megavoltage irradiation and conventional intracavitary techniques at the M.D. Anderson between the years of 1954 and 1963. A comparable recurrence rate (33%, 72/218), was reported for similar patients treated at the same institution between 1964 and 1969 [26], implying that no improvement in local control rates had been accomplished during those 15 years. Kolstad [27], in a recent review of stage IIIB patients treated at the Norwegian Radium Hospital, found that results have remained constant during the last 40 years (1933–1975), despite technological improvements and a better understanding of tumor radiobiology.

The 23.8% pelvic failure rate in our patients represents marked improvement over the 36% to 53% local recurrence rate reported by other investigators using conventional intracavitary techniques [14, 15, 24–27]. Whether the improved local tumor control rates will translate into improved survival remains to be seen. However, recent reports from the University of Maryland showed a significant improvement in both, local control and survival, in patients with stage IIIB disease treated with interstitial implants [6, 7].

There is little information in the literature about the influence that clinical and radiological findings may have on local failure rates in stage IIIB cancer of the cervix. It has been observed that patients with tumor fixation to both pelvic walls, and/or extension into distal vagina, and those with bilateral hydronephrosis have low survival rates [25, 26, 28]. It is not clear however, whether the poor prognosis is the result of failure to control the pelvic tumor or metastatic spread or both.

Local failure rates are not usually analyzed as a function of unilateral or bilateral pelvic wall fixation. In this respect, the staging classification used at the M.D. Anderson Hospital is very useful since stage III patients are subdivided into IIIA and IIIB, according to unilateral or bilateral pelvic wall fixation. Our results in patients with unilateral pelvic wall fixation (20.6% local recurrence) compare favorably with the 28.7% pelvic failure rate reported in similar patients from that institution. The pelvic failure rate in patients with bilateral pelvic wall fixation utilizing conventional intracavitary applicators is unacceptably high [25–27]. As illustrated in Table 7, a substantial improvement in pelvic failure rates is seen in patients who pre-

Table 7. Bilateral pelvic-wall fixation versus pelvic failure.

Institution	No. cases	Pelvic failure
Princess Margaret		(57.0%) [a]
M.D. Anderson	333	151/333 (45.0%) [a]
Univ. of Arizona	6	3/6 (50.0%) [a]
	21	7/21 (33.0%) [b]

[a] Standard intracavitary technique.
[b] Interstitial parametrial implant.

sented with bilateral pelvic wall fixation and were treated with the interstitial implants; the local recurrence was reduced from 45%–57% to 33%.

Similarly, the presence of hydronephrosis has been associated with lower survival but, no information about the sites of failure is given [30]. The pelvic recurrence rate in our patients with no evidence of ureteral obstruction was quite similar to the failure rate seen in patients with unilateral hydronephrosis (22% and 18% respectively). Patients with bilateral hydronephrosis on the other hand, had a significantly higher risk for local recurrence (75%). This finding strongly suggest, that a more vigorous approach, either with radiation alone or a combination of radiation and chemotherapy, regional hyperthermia or both, is warranted in these patients.

The presence of residual tumor at the time of the intracavitary radium, a common finding in patients with advanced disease, has important prognostic implications. Grossman and coworkers [23], reported a significantly better prognosis for patients with stage III cervical cancer who had optimal tumor response than in those who responded poorly to external radiation. Tak *et al.* [15], found that 87% of patients with residual tumor at the time of the radium application, died of the disease, most of them with persistent or recurrent tumor in the pelvis. They concluded that the most important factor in local failure was the volume of residual tumor at the time of the radium application.

The findings in our study (Table 4) not only confirmed the predictive value of tumor regression assessed at the time of the implant procedure, but also attest to the efficacy of the interstitial implant in controlling disease in patients who experienced complete or partial tumor regression. In contrast, patients who did not demonstrate some tumor response during the external radiation course, are at high risk for local failure (75%). They should also be considered for new therapeutic strategies such as a combination of radiation with either regional hyperthermia or with chemotherapy or both [28].

In other series [24], patients who present with distorted anatomy from gross residual tumor and/or narrow vaults were not considered for placement of intrauterine tandem and vaginal ovoids and then are suboptimally treated with external irradiation alone. In our series, despite the fact that distorted anatomy was present in many patients, all underwent the implant procedure. This constitutes another important advantage of the interstitial implant technique over the intracavitary approach.

Complications

At the beginning of our experience, it was common practice to insert obturator needles on the surface of the vaginal obturator, and to load them with radioactive sources. Because of the active length selected (6 cm), the more distal 2–3 cm of the active portion of the sources protruded into the upper vagina. This concentric configuration of the implant led to the upper wall of the vagina being sandwiched circumferentially between the protruding sources on the surface of the obturator and the next concentric row of loaded needles. This central 'hot spot' and the proximity of the sources to the vaginal mucosa, explains not only the high frequency, but also the nature of the complications seen in our early experience. Of seven patients treated in this fashion, six (86%), developed severe complications, five of them had recto or vesicovaginal fistula, or both (seven fistulae in five patients).

This observation prompted us to stop using the needsles on the surface of the vaginal cylinder when a uterine tandem was in place. If a tandem could not be utilized the central needles are inserted and loaded with shorter active length microsources (4 cm instead of 6 cm A.L.). Since our early data also suggested that the aspects of the milligram-hours and its distribution played an important role in the development of complications, the total milligram-hours was limited to a maximum of 5000, and modifications in implant geometry were implemented.

These changes results in a marked reduction of the incidence and severity of complications in the remaining patients. This reduction in morbidity was accomplished without a reduction in the primary control of pelvic disease [29].

Conclusions

On the basis of this study we believe the following conclusions about transperineal interstitial irradiation to parametria in cancer of the cervix stage IIB and IIIB are warranted:

1. The procedure is safe: no fatal complications have occurred and with the modifications described, the frequency and severity of radiation side effects has been reduced to acceptable levels.

2. It is effective: pelvic control rates particularly in stage IIIB are high, irrespective of tumor size, fixation to one or both pelvic walls, or extent of vaginal disease. In stage IIB, continued use of parametrial implants is justified in selected groups of patients: in patients with gross residual tumor at the time of the brachytherapy application. On the other hand, interstitial implants do not appear to be a satisfactory substitute for extrafascial hysterectomy in patients with 'barrel shaped' lesions.
3. It has a wider applicability and greater flexibility than conventional intracavitary applicators particularly in patients with distorted anatomy.

Acknowledgements

The author is indebted to Drs Valencia and Ocampo for their collaboration work and to Ms Esneda Canizales for her invaluable assistance with the follow-up of the patients. Ms Leslie Pike is thanked for typing the manuscript.

References

1. Griffith G (ed). 1968. Cooperative international studies in epidemiology of cancer. Cancer Management, Lippincott Co, Philadelphia.
2. Correa P, Llenos G. 1966. Morbidity and mortality from cancer in Cali, Colombia. J Natl Cancer Inst 36:717–745.
3. Silverberg E. 1979. Cancer statistics, 1979. Cancer 29:6–21.
4. Arneson AN. 1938. Use of interstitial radiation in the treatment of cancer of the cervix. Radiology 30:167–179.
5. Pitts HC, Waterman GW. 1940. Further report on the radium treatment of carcinoma of the cervix uteri. Am J Roentgenol 43:567–571.
6. Prempree T, Scott RM. 1978. Treatment of stage III-B carcinoma of the cervix. Improvement in local by radium needle implant to supplement the dose to the parametrium. Cancer 412:1105–1113.
7. Prempree T. 1983. Parametrial implant in stage III-B cancer of the cervix. A five year study. Cancer 52:748-750.
8. Feder BH, Syed AMN, Neblett D. 1978. Treatment of extensive carcinoma of the cervix with the 'transperineal parametrial butterfly'. Int J Radiat Oncol Biol Phys 4:735–742.
9. Aristizabal SA, Surwit EA, Hevezi JM, Heusinkveld RS. 1983. Treatment of advanced cancer of the cervix with transperineal interstitial irradiation. Int J Radiat Oncol Biol Phys 9:1013–1017.
10. Aristizabal SA, Valancia A, Surwit EA, Hevezi JM. 1983. Treatment of locally advanced cancer of the cervix with transperineal interstitial irradiation. Report on 106 cases. Am J Clin Oncol 6:645–650.
11. Combes PF, Daly NJ, Horiot JC, Achille E, Keiling R, Pigneux J, Pourquier H, Rozan R, Schraub S, Vrousos C. 1985. Results of radiotherapy alone in 581 patients with stage II carcinoma of the uterine cervix. 11:463–471.

12. Durrance FY, Fletcher GH, Rutledge FN. 1969. Analysis of central recurrent disease in stage I and II squamous cell carcinomas of the cervix on intact uterus. Am J Roentgenol. :831-838.
13. Montana GS. 1985. Analysis of results of radiation therapy for stage II carcinoma of the cervix. Cancer 55:956–962.
14. Perez C, Breaux S, Madoc-Jones H, Bedwinek JM, Camel HM, Purdy JA, Walz BJ. 1983. Radiation therapy alone in the treatment of carcinoma of uterine cervix. I. Analysis of tumor recurrence. Cancer 51:1393–1402.
15. Tak WK, Munzendrider JE, Mitchell GW. 1979. External irradiation and one radium application for carcinoma of the cervix. Int J Radiat Oncol Biol Phys 5:29–36.
16. Lu T, Macasaet MA, Nelson JH. 1976. The barrel shaped cervical carcinoma. Am J Obstet Gynecol 124:596–600.
17. O'Quinn AG, Fletcher GH, Wharton JT. 1980. Guidelines for conservative hysterectomy after irradiation. Gynecol Oncol 9:68–79.
18. Perez CA, Bedwinek JM, Kao MS. 1983. Carcinoma of the uterine cervix, significance of barrel-shaped configuration in stage I-B, II-A, and II-B. Proceedings of the 25th Annual ASTR Meeting 9:85.
19. Nelson AJ, Fletcher GH, Wharton JT. 1975. Indication for adjunctive conservative extra-fascial hysterectomy in selected cases of carcinoma of the uterine cervix. Am J Roentgenol Rad Nucl Med 123:91–99.
20. Mendenhall WM, Thar TL, Bova FJ, Marcus RB, Morgan LS, Million RR. 1984. Prognositic and treatment factors affecting pelvic control of stage IB and IIA-B carcinoma of the intact uterine cervix treated with radiation therapy alone. Cancer 53:2649–2654.
21. Van Nagell JR, Rayburn W, Donaldson ES, Hanson M, Gay EC, Yoneda J, Maruyuma Y, Powell DF. 1979. Therapeutic implications of patterns of recurrence in cancer of the uterine cervix. Cancer 44:2354–2362.
22. Hardt N, Van Nagell SR, Hanson M, Donalson E, Yoneda S, Maruyama Y. 1982. Radiation induced tumor regression as a prognostic factor in patients with invasive cervical cancer. Cancer 49:35–39.
23. Grossman I, Kurohara SS, Webster JH, George FW. 1973. The prognostic significance of tumor response during radiotherapy in cervical carcinoma. Radiology 107:411–415.
24. Montana GS, Fowler WE, Mahesh AV, Walton LA, Mack Y, Shemanski L. Carcinoma of cervix stage III. Accepted for publication in Cancer.
25. Paunier JP, Delclos L, Fletcher GH. 1967. Causes, time of death and sites of failure in squamous cell carcinoma of the uterine cervix on intact uterus. Radiology 88:555–562.
26. Jampolis S, Sandras EJ, Fletcher GH. 1975. Analysis of sites and causes of failures of irradiation in invasive squamous cell carcinoma of the intact uterine cervix. Radiology 115:681–685.
27. Kolstad P. 1983. Value and complications of periaortic irradiation in advanced cervical cancer. In: Recent clinical developments in gynecologic oncology. (Paul Morrow *et al,* ed). Raven Press, New York.
28. Thomas G, Dembo A, Beale F, Bean H, Bush R, Herman J, Pringle J, Gayle R, Sturgeon J, Fine S, Black B. 1984. Concurrent radiation, Mitomycin C and 5-Fluorouracil in poor prognosis carcinoma of cervix: Preliminary results of a phase I-II study. Int J Radiat Oncol Biol Phys 10:1785–1790.
29. Aristizabal S, Valencia A, Ocampo G, Surwit E. 1985. Interstitial parametrial irradiation in cancer of the cervix stage IIB-IIIB. Analysis of pelvic control and complications. Endocurietherapy/Hyperthermia Oncol 1:41–48.
30. Bosch A, Frias Z, DeValda G. 1973. Prognostic significance of ureteral obstruction in carcinoma of the cervix uteri. Acta Radiol 12:47–55.

8. Hydroxyurea and radiation therapy in the treatment of carcinoma of the cervix

M. STEVEN PIVER

Notwithstanding the marked improvement in radiation technology over the past decades, the survival rates of patients with cervical cancer who receive this therapy remains unsatisfactory. It is clear that fewer women are dying from cervical cancer, however, this is not related to improved therapy for invasive cervical cancer. Rather, the significant decrease in the death rate is a direct result of the lower incidence of invasive cervical cancer related to the Papanicolau smear which allows for the diagnosis of cervical cancer in an *in situ* stage. In support of this contention that improved radiation technological advances have not led to concomitant increase in survival, are the 5-year survival rates utilizing kilavoltage as compared to megavoltage radiation equipment as reported by Fletcher and Rutledge [1]. As seen in Table 1, the radiotherapy results for stage IIB and IIIB cervical cancer did not improve from the change from kilavoltage (1948–1954) and megavoltage (1954–1963) time periods.

Since improved technology did not result in improved survival, other explanations were sought. A decade ago it was discovered that a significant number of patients with locally advanced cervical cancer (stage IIB-IV) never had the entire cancer radiated. Specifically, of our first 100 patients with FIGO stage IIB, IIIB and IV cervical cancer who underwent pretherapy surgical staging para-aortic lymphadenectomy or para-aortic node biopsy,

Table 1. Squamous cell carcinoma of the cervic; 5-year survival rate.

Stage	Kilavoltage 1948–1954 (%)	Megavoltage 1954–1963 (%)
II B	60.0	66.5
III B	31.0	36.0
IV	5.0	14.0

Fletcher and Rutledge [1].

E.A. Surwit, D.S. Alberts (eds) Cervix Cancer.

13% of the stage IIB, 36% of the stage IIIB and 57% of the stage IV patients had histologic confirmation of para-aortic node metastasis ... out of the field of pelvic radiation [2].

Thus, treatment of the entire extent of the malignancy became axiomatic. Because of the intolerance of the normal pelvic tissues, bladder, rectum, and terminal ileum to increasing doses of radiation, there became a need for agents that would potentiate the killing effect of irradiation of tumor cells without a concomitant increase in the damage to the normal pelvic structures. Before Hydroxyurea (HU) was considered as a possible radiation sensitizer, it was looked on as a possible chemotherapeutic agent. First synthesized in 1869 by Dresler and Stein [3], however, it was not until 1928 when HU was found by Rosenthal and co-authors [4] to produce anemia, severe leukopenia and megoblastic changes of the peripheral blood and bone marrow ... clearly, properties to be exploited against tumor cells. In the sixties reports documented that HU was effective against squamous cell cancers, adenocarcinomas, melanomas, sarcomas, and chronic leukemia but had found little use as a chemotherapeutic agent because its daily administration led to the development of severe megoblastic anemia unresponsive to therapy [5, 6]. However, in 1965 a report by Lerner and Beckloff [7] suggested that HU administered intermittently, at a dose of 80 mg/kg every 3 days, reduced toxicity without concomitant decrease in antitumor effect and thus might qualify as a chemotherapeutic agent.

At this point in time there were no considerations for combining HU and radiation therapy as a potential radiation sensitizer. However, in 1964 Young [8] reported that HU directly inhibited DNA synthesis without effecting the synthesis of RNA or protein in *in vitro* tissue cultures. Subsequent studies by Sinclair [9] provided the basis for expecting that HU would sensitize mammalian cells to the effects of radiation. Sinclair demonstrated that HU selectively killed cells that were synthezising DNA (S phase of the cell cycle) at concentrations that had no killing effect on cells in other phases of the cell cycle. He demonstrated that G1 (postmitotic) and G2 (premitotic) stages in the cell cycle of the Chinese hampsters are more radiosensitive than the S phase (DNA synthetic period) [10]. His studies showed that HU preferentially killed S phase cells while G1 and G2 cells were apparently not effected. G1 phase cells did not progress into S phase, but-were blocked at the G1/S interphase. Cells in G2 appeared to progress through mitosis into the G1/S stage without delay. Consequently, HU would act to destroy the relatively radioresistent cells in S phase and block the surviving cells at the G1/S interphase, a relatively radiosensitive portion of the cell cycle. Further, his results were of special interest in that G1 cells were most sensitive to the actions of x-ray radiation and that the combination of HU plus X-ray radiation resulted in increased cell kill as compared to X-ray radiation alone (Figure 1).

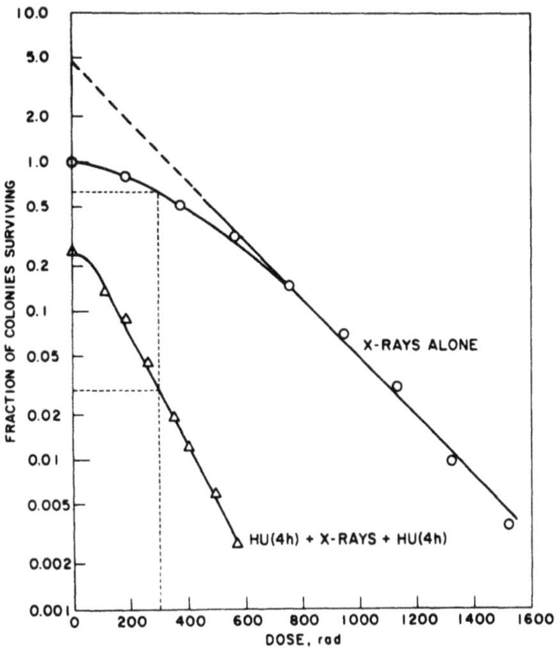

Figure 1. Survival curves in animal cells for X-rays alone and for X-rays in cells pretreated and posttreated with Hydroxyurea (HU), showing HU use requires fewer rads (reprinted with permission).

Thus, there are several mechanisms by which HU is used in combination with radiation therapy and could be of benefit. First, by syncronization of cells within the mitotic cycle in a radiation sensitive portion of the cycle. As stated, HU has been shown to destroy the relatively radioresistant cells synthesizing DNA (S phase) and to cause the surviving cells in the relatively radiosensitive G1/S interphase. The net result of HU would be to inactivate the resistant cells and to sensitize the remaining cells. A second mechanism of action would be an agent which would prevent the repair of cells from sublethal radiation damage. Phillips and Tolmach [11] have demonstrated that HU prevents the repair of sublethally damaged cells by radiation. Thus, the continued use of HU after completion of radiation would not allow sublethally damaged cervical cancer cells to repair and repopulate the tumor. Thirdly, many radiation therapy failures are in large tumors containing many hypoxic cells. With the reduction of the size of the tumor by the killing action of fractionated radiation on the aerobic cells, there is improvement in the vascularization of the tumor. Many of the hypoxic cells (G0) then become aerobic, enter the expanded aerobic cell cycle allowing HU to inactivate the S phase cells and syncronizing the remaining cells at the G1/S interphase. Thus, it is therefore theoretically possible that HU has the following actions: (1) destroys cells that are in the radioresistant part of the cycle; (2) syncronize the remaining cells that are in the radiosensitive por-

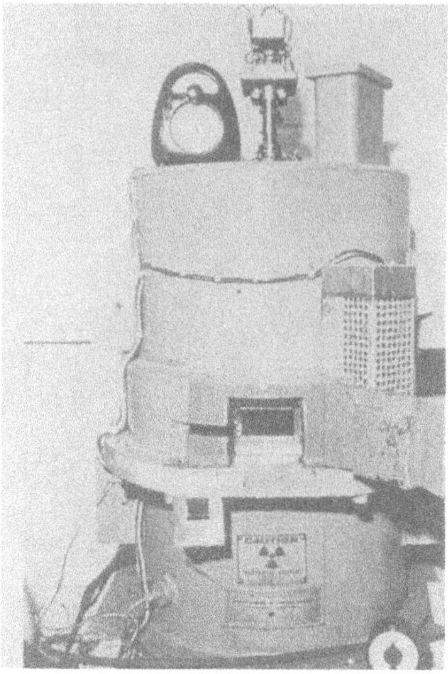

Figure 2. Cesium 137 use for radiation plus Hydroxyurea experiments in mice.

tion of the mitotic cycle; (3) prevent repair of the sublethally radiation damaged cells; (4) shrinkage of the tumor to improve vascularization allowing for hypoxic cells to enter the aerobic cycle and proliferate and are thus subject to the effect of HU.

The *in vitro* study of Sinclair [10] and the clinical studies of Lerner *et al.* [12] utilize HU and radiation in locally advanced cancers of the head and neck stimulated our interest in the combination of HU and radiation and prompted a series of experiments employing an animal tumor system [13], since there were no such studies in lower animals with the ultimate goal to use this combination in women with locally advanced cervical cancer.

Third-generation isotransplants of a spontaneous C3H-HE mouse mammary carcinoma were employed. Transplants were made from cell suspensions prepared from freshly excised second generation isotransplants; the latter were derived from first generation isotransplant tissue which had been maintained in liquid nitrogen. An inoculum of 5–10 μl os suspension containing $5–10 \times 10^5$ viable tumor cells was injected into the muscle of the mouses leg.

Treatment was performed using a specially designed cesium 137 unit which featured two opposed sources and a treatment field of 50 cm diameter (Figure 2). Treatment conditions had been designated: (1) *Hypoxia* (application of a heavy clamp across the route of the thigh 2 min prior to radiation); (2) *air* (the animal respiring air at 1 atmosphere of pressure); (3) *high*

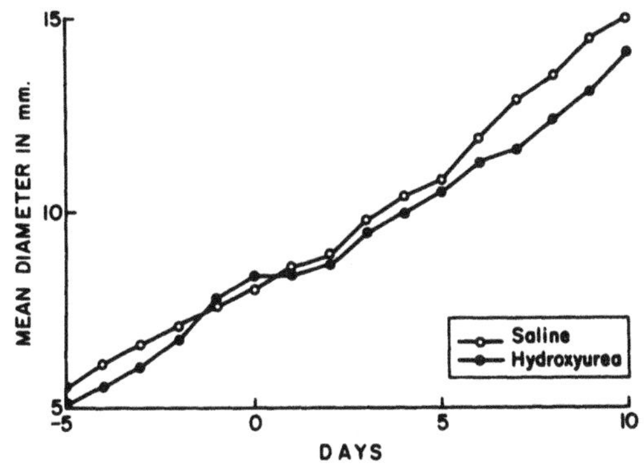

Figure 3. The growth of tumors in mice injected with either a single hydroxyurea (LD1) dose or saline. Hydroxyurea produced no delay in tumor growth (reprinted with permission).

pressure oxygen (the animal respiring pure oxygen in three atmospheres of pressure for 5 min during local radiation).

Radiation was begun when the mean of three diameters reached a value of 8+ - 0–5 mm, i.e. a tumor volume of approximately 250 mm^3. At weekly intervals after treatment the tumor was scored ± for presence of recurrent tumor. When the diameter of the recurrent tumor was 12 mm the animal was sacrificed and lungs were examined grossly for the presence of metastasis. Mice surviving for 120 days without recurrence were scored as having locally controlled tumors, at which time their lungs were examined for the presence of tumor metastasis. At the end point of each assay is the TCD 50 or the radiation dose which on the average would be expected to prevent recurrence of the irradiated tumors in one-half of the mice for the time specified.

To be certain that Hu at the dosage employed did not have a significant tumor inhibiting effect of its own, the growth of tumors in mice injected with either single HU doses or with saline without radiation therapy was studied. As in Figure 3, HU injected produced no delay in tumor growth as compared to saline.

Table 2. Multidose Hydroxyurea and fractionated radiation CS-137; C_3H mammary carcinoma.

	TCD 50/rads		
Radiation condition	Saline	Hydroxyurea*	Differential rads
Hypoxia	11,340	9980	1360
Air	7,500	6632	868
Hyperbaric oxygen	4,500	3912	588

* 2 g/kg every third day; 262 mice; Piver *et al.* [13].

In the multidose radiation studies five equal radiation fractions 72 h between each fraction were administered. In this instance HU was given in 13 injections with 72 h between injections. HU was started 72 h before the first radiation and continued for 21 days after the final irradiation does. HU was administered 2 h before each irradiation. Two-hundred and sixty-two tumors were studied. One-half received HU and the other half saline. As seen in Table 2 it required 1360, 868, 588 less rads of radiation under hypoxic, air or hyperbaric oxygen conditions respectively for mice who received HU as compared to saline.

Thus having demonstrated the potentiating effect of HU on radiation in tumor in lower animals, we began in the early 1970s to evaluate the possible radiation potentiating effects of HU in women with locally advanced carcinoma of the uterine cervix. Our first prospective randomized double blind study in women with locally advanced cervical cancer was carried out in 1971 [14]. This included 37 women with stage IIB and IIIB cervical cancer none of whom underwent pretherapy surgical (para-aortic node biopsy) staging. For the stage IIB patients, 46.1% in the placebo group were NED at 2 years as compared to 77.7% in the HU group ($p = 0.003$). Of the stage IIIB patients 11% (one of nine) in the placebo group were NED at 2 years as compared to 50% (three of six) who received HU ($p = 0.3$). Of the total women that received HU 66.6% (10/15) were NED at 2 years versus 31.8% (7/22) of the placebo group ($p = 0.001$) (Table 3).

After completion of our initial randomized study in 37 women with stage IIB and IIIB cervical carcinoma it became evident that with the advent of surgical staging by exploratory laparotomy and para-aortic lymphadenectomy at out institute [15], that a significant number of patients with clinical stage IIB and IIIB cervical cancer had metastasis beyond the field of pelvic irradiation, i.e. metastasis to the para-aortic lymph nodes. Therefore, with the advent of surgical staging, two prospective randomized trials were initiated to compare HU and placebo in women with cervical cancer. In our second report 130 evaluable women with stage IIIB and IIIB cervical cancer were randomly assigned to receive HU or placebo and megavoltage radiation therapy.

Table 3. Two-year survival without evidence of cervical cancer.

Stage	Hydroxyurea (%)	Placebo (%)	p-value
IIB	77.7	46.1	0.03
IIIB	50.0	11.1	0.13
Total	66.6	31.8	0.0014

Piver *et al.* [14].

Of the patients with stage IIB cervical cancer without biopsy proof of aortic node metastasis (staged and non-staged), a significant improvement in survival (p = 0.01) was achieved in the HU group (74.0%) as compared to the patients who received placebo (42.5%). There was a trend towards improved survival in HU patients with stage IIIB disease without biopsy proof (staged and non-staged) of aortic node metastasis as compared to the patients who received placebo which did not reach statistical (p = 0.22) significance: HU group (52.1%) as compared to the placebo group (33.3%) (Tabble 4).

Our third study was a prospective double blind study in which HU was compared to placebo in patients with FIGO stage IIB cervical cancer in which all patients underwent pretherapy para-aortic lymphadenectomy and were found to be without histopathologic evidence of metastasis to the para-aortic nodes [16]. From June 1972 to December 1976, 40 patients with FIGO stage IIB cervical carcinoma were entered into a prospective double blind randomized study to evaluate the possible radiation potentiating properties of HU, i.e. improved survival. All patients were documented to be without aortic lymph node metastasis by pretherapy staging para-aortic lymphadenectomy. All patients were followed for longer than 5 years (5.2–9.2 years) or until death. The double blind code was not broken until all patients had been followed for a minimum of 2–5 years. Life table survival for the patients given HU was 94% as compared to 53% for patients given placebo (p = 0.001) (Figure 4). Only one (5%) patient given HU died of cervical cancer. Of the other patients who died in the group given HU, all were confirmed by postmortem examination to have been without recurrent cervical cancer. In contrast, 45% (nine) of the patients given placebo died of cervical cancer.

Radiation sensitizers are of clinical value if there is a significant differential between the effect on tumor as compared to that on normal cells. In the current study, this was evident. There was no adverse reaction on the skin within the radiated area in either the HU or placebo group. The intestine was not sensitized during radiationtherapy, as evidenced by the degree of severe diarrhea in both the HU and placebo group (p = 0.47). Moreover,

Table 4. Two-year survival without evidence of cervical cancer.

Stage	Hydroxyurea (%)	Placebo (%)	p-value
II B	74	42	0.01
III B	52	33	NS
Total	64	39	

Piver *et al.* [15].

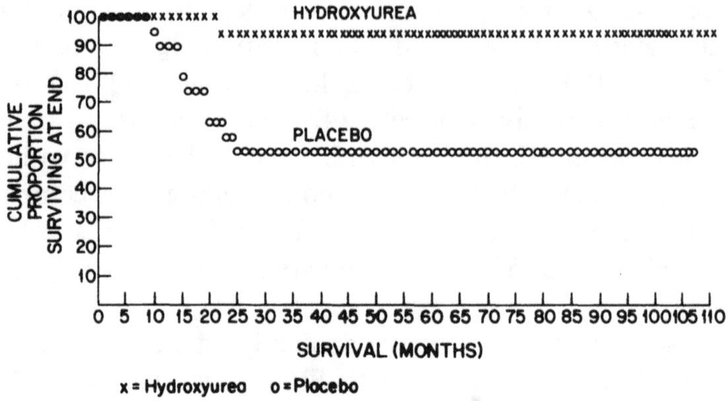

Figure 4. Duration of survival of all patients (40) with stage IIB cervical cancer (reprinted with permission).

there were more radiation complications that required surgical correction in the patients given placebo than the patients given HU ($p = 0.50$). There was no significant anemia or thrombocytopenia in either group. However, 16 of 20 patients in the HU group developed leukopenia as compared to three of 20 in the placebo group ($p = 0.001$).

In this study we were concerned about the high rate of radiation complications in both patients given HU and those given placebo. Many of the complications with staging para-aortic lymphadenectomy in women with carcinoma of the uterine cervix were related to the type of incision and subsequent use of external radiation. Transperitoneal staging para-aortic lymphadenectomy frequently results in sections of the ileum or jejunum adhering to the undersurface of the incision and thereby restricting the normal mobility of the intestine. This process results in a higher dose of radiation to the adherent segment of small intestine and leads to possible obstruction and/or development of a fistula. However, the use of retroperitoneal incision for staging para-aortic lymphadenectomy may significantly decrease these complications [17].

Notwithstanding the outstanding survival results in our stage IIB cervical cancer patients who were surgically staged and received HU plus pelvic radiation, it was apparent that the vast majority of patients with stage IIB carcinoma of the uterine cervix do not undergo pretherapy surgical staging para-aortic lymphadenectomy prior to pelvic radiation. Therefore, a fourth study was carried out to evaluate the survival rates of patients with stage IIB cervical cancer treated with pelvic radiation plus HU who did not undergo pretherapy para-aortic lymphadenectomy but who had a negative pretherapy bipedal lymphangiogram [18]. We assumed that in those patients who did not undergo pretherapy staging para-aortic lymphadenectomy, a pretherapy negative bipedal lymphangiogram might be clinically useful in elim-

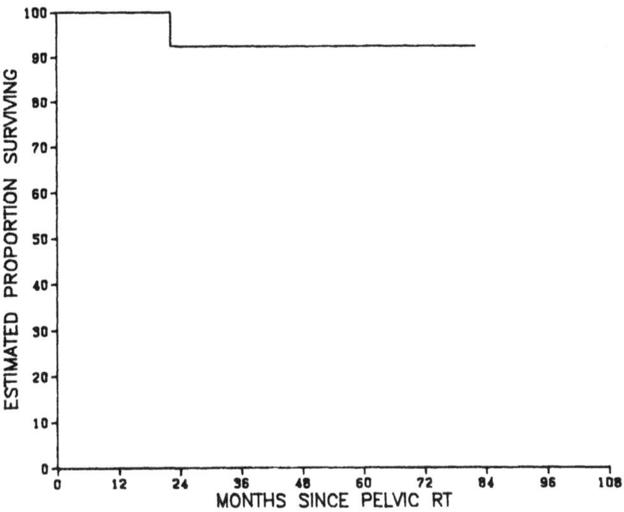

Figure 5. Disease-free survival rate in 20 non-surgically staged patients with negative lymphangiograms who had stage IIB carcinoma of the cervix treated by pelvic radiation plus Hyroxyurea (reprinted with permission).

inating most of those who had metastasis outside of the field of pelvic radiation to the para-aortic lymph nodes. This assumption was based on our previous report on 103 patients with cervical cancer who underwent lymphangiography followed by biopsy of the retroperitoneal lymph nodes [19]. With the use of strict criteria of metastasis to the lymph nodes, a filling defect in the lymph nodes not transversed by lymphatics, a positive biopsy confirmed the diagnosis of metastatic disease in 41 of 42 patients (97%). Of the 61 patients who had lymphagiograms that were read as negative for metastasis, 12 (19%) had positive lymph node biopsy. A false negative rate is accounted for by the fact that a metastasis that is less than 3 mm in diameter will not cause a defect in the lymph nodes significant enough to be detected by roentgenographic examination. Secondly, all pelvic and para-aortic lymph nodes are not filled by the contrast materials. These two factors explain why a roentgenogram could be read as negative and a subsequent biopsy could be performed.

From 1977 to 1984 20 patients fulfilled the criteria of (1) FIGO stage IIB, (2) histologically documented cervical cancer, (3) had negative bipedal lymphangiogram reviewed by the senior author (MSP), (4) pelvic radiation, (5) HU, (6) no staging laparotomy and (7) no surgical procedure as part of the initial treatment [20]. The treatment plan was to deliver approximately 5040 rads over 5 weeks followed by 3500 to 4000 rads to point A by intracavitary and vaginal radium in one or two applications. The median dose for the 20 patients was 5020 rads (4000–5040) of external radiation. All patients received intrauterine and vaginal radium for a median dose of 4000 rads to point A (1500–5000 rads). The toxicity was not dissimilar to our previous studies. No patient developed severe skin reaction. Severe diarrhea occurred in 20%, 15% developed anemia, 85% leukopenia but no patient developed thrombocytopenia. Of the 20 patients, three (15%) developed complications requiring surgical intervention. The estimated 5-year survival rate was 92% and the estimated 5-year disease free survival rate was 88% (Figure 5). 17 patients were alive with no evidence of disease with a median follow-up of 28 months (6–83), one patient died of intercurrent disease with no evidence of disease at 17 months with a thrombosed abdominal aorta, one patient is alive with no evidence of disease (18 months after recurrence to the chest wall) and one patient died of cervical cancer 22 months after recurrence to the para-aortic nodes. Neither patient developed a recurrence within the irradiated area.

Our most recent report was of patients with stage IIIB cervical carcinoma who underwent pretherapy surgical staging para-aortic lymphadenectomy and were randomized in a double blind fashion to HU plus pelvic radiation or pelvic radiation plus placebo [20]. There were 45 evaluable patients with stage IIIB carcinoma of the uterine cervix entered into this study. All patients were documented to be without para-aortic lymph node metastasis by pretherapy staging para-aortic lymphadenectomy.

The initial plan of therapy was for continuous therapy (200 rads/day) or 6000 rads of pelvic radiation in 6 weeks plus intrauterine radiation. However, 16 patients incorrectly received 6000 rads pelvic radiation in 8 weeks by split course therapy (2 weeks rest after 3000 rads) plus radium. Twenty-nine patients received the planned continuous therapy of 6000 rads in 6 weeks plus radium. The median dose of pelvic radiation in patients who received continuous therapy or split course therapy radiation was 6000 rads. Leukopenia ($\leq 2500/mm^3$) was significantly increased in patients given HU as compared to those given placebo ($p = 0.001$). There was no statistically significant difference in toxicity relative to anemia, thrombocytopenia, radiation skin reaction, diarrhea, or radiation induced complications requiring surgical correction. The estimated 5-year progression free survival rates in the combined, continuous and split course radiation therapy patients was 60 and 52% for the corresponding placebo patients ($p = 0.49$). However, the 5-year progression free survival rates for the correctly treated patients (continuous therapy of 6000 rads in 6 weeks) was 91% for the HU group and 60% for the placebo group ($p = 0.06$) (Figure 6).

In 1979 the Gynecologic Oncology Group Study reported the use of HU and radiation therapy in stage IIIB and IV cervical cancer. Of 104 patients randomly assigned to radiation with HU or placebo, without prior surgical staging para-aortic lymphadenectomy, survival and progression free interval was significantly better in patients who received HU plus pelvic radiation as

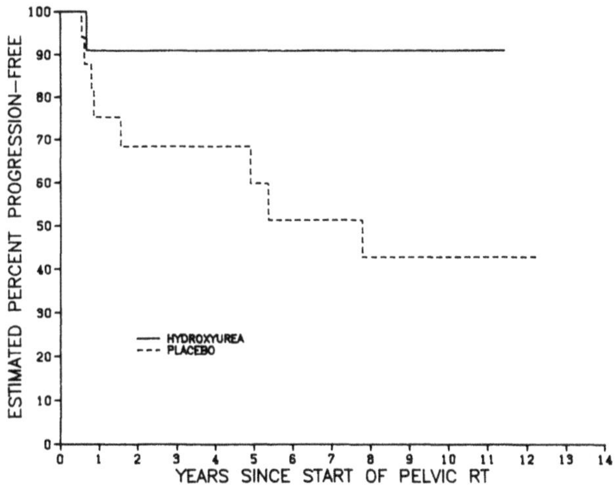

Figure 6. Stage IIIB carcinoma cervix negative para-aortic lymphadenectomy continuous course pelvic radiation (reprinted with permission).

compared to placebo plus pelvic radiation [21]. To date, they have not reported results in surgically staged patients.

The very high survival rates of 94% at 5 years in surgically stages patients (negative para-aortic lymph nodes) with stage IIB cervical cancer, the 92% estimated 5-year survival of non-surgically staged patients with negative bipedal lymphangiogram (negative pelvic and para-aortic lymph nodes) who had stage IIB cervical cancer, and the 91% estimated 5-year survival in surgically staged patients with stage IIIB cervical cancer, all of whom were treated with Hydroxyurea plus pelvic radiation, without significant adverse effects on the normal tissues, suggests that HU is indeed a significant radiation potentiator.

References

1. Fletcher GH, Rutledge RN. 1967. Overall results in radiotherapy in carcinoma of the cervix. Clin Obstet Gynecol 10:958.
2. Piver MS. 1977. Value of pretherapy para-aortic lymphadenectomy for carcinoma of the cervix uteri. Surg Gynecol Obstet 145:17.
3. Dressler WFC, Stein R, 1869. Ueber den Hydroxylharnstoff. Ann Chemie 150:242.
4. Rosenthal F, Wislicki I, Kollek L. 1928. Ueber die Beziehungen von schwersten Blutgiften zu Abbauprodukten des Eiweisses. Beitrag zum Enstehungsmechanismus derperniziosen Anamie. Klin Wochenschr 7:972.
5. Thurman WG. 1964. Pharmacology and antitumor effect of Hydroxyurea (abstract). Proc Am Assoc Cancer Res 4:67.
6. Stearns B, Losee KA, Bertstein J. 1963. Hydroxyurea: new type of potential antitumor agent. J Med Chem 6:201.
7. Lerner HJ, Beckloff GL. 1965. Hydroxyurea administered intermittently. JAMA 192:138.

8. Young CW, Hodas S. 1964. Hydroxyurea: inhibitory effect on DNA metabolism. Science 146:1172.
9. Sinclair WK. 1965. Hydroxyurea: differential lethal efects on cultured mammilian cells during the cell cycle. Science 150:1729.
10. Sinclair WK. 1968. The combined effect of Hydroxyurea and X-rays in Chinese hamster cells in vitro. Cancer Res 28:190.
11. Phillips RA, Tolmach IJ. 1966. Repair of potentially lethal damage in x-irradiated HeLa cells. Radiat Res 29:413.
12. Lerner HJ, Beckloff GL, Godwin MD. 1969. Concomitant Hydroxyurea and radiotherapy in the management of 60 patients with head and neck cancer. Am Surg 35:525–534.
13. Piver MS, Howes AE, Suite HD *et al.* 1972. Effect of hydroxyurea on the radiation response of C3H mouse mammary tumors. Cancer 29:407.
14. Piver MS, Barlow JJ, Vongtama V *et al.* 1974. Hydroxyurea and radiation therapy in advanced cervical cancer. Am J Obstet Gynecol 120:969.
15. Piver MS, Barlow JJ, Vontama V. 1977. Hydroxyurea as a radiation sensitizer in women with carcinoma of the uterine cervix. Am J Obstet Gynecol 129:379.
16. Piver MS, Barlow JJ, Vongtama V *et al.* 1983. Hydroxyurea. A radiation potentiator in carcinoma of the uterine cervix. A randomized double blind study. Am J Obstet Gynecol 147:803.
17. Berman ML, Lagasse LD, Watring WG *et al.* 1977. The operative evaluation of patients with cervical carcinoma by an extraperitoneal approach. Obstet Gynecol 50:658.
18. Piver MS, Krishnamsetty R, Emrich L. 1985. Survival of non-surgically staged patients with negative lymphangiogram Stage IIB carcinoma of the cervix treated by pelvic radiation plus Hydroxyurea. Am J Obstet Gynecol 151:1006.
19. Piver MS, Wallace S, Castro JR 1971. The accuracy of lymphangiography in carcinoma of the uterine cervix. Am J Roent Rad Ther Nucl Med 111:278–283.
20. Piver MS, Vongtama V, Emrich LJ. 1985. Hydroxyurea plus pelvic radiation versus placebo plus pelvic radiation in surgically staged stage IIIB cervical cancer. J Surg Oncol (in press).
21. Hreshchyshyn MM, Aron BS, Boronow RC *et al.* 1979. Hydroxyurea of placebo combined with radiation to treat Stage IIIB and IV cervical cancer confined to the pelvis. Int J Radiat Oncol Biol Phys 5:317.

9. Single agent chemotherapy in carcinoma of the cervix

J. TATE THIGPEN

Introduction

The incidence of invasive cancer of the cervix has decreased dramatically since 1950 as a result of the widespread use of screening with the PAP smear. Despite this success, estimates for 1986 still predict 14,000 new cases of invasive disease with 6,800 deaths [1]. While a majority of invasive cases are treated initially with surgery and/or radiotherapy, the number of deaths indicates that a significant proportion will recur or will present with disseminated disease initially and thus be candidates for systemic therapy. In addition, those patients with locally advanced disease and a high risk for recurrence are now being evaluated for adjuvant therapy with systemic agents. The need to identify active agents for such therapy is thus evident. This discussion will focus on studies of single drugs in patients with advanced or recurrent carcinoma of the cervix.

General considerations

Prior to 1976, carcinoma of the cervix was studied primarily as a part of broader phase II trials [2]. Data on agent activity were derived from compilation of cases from a number of sources. These data were fraught with the problems of non-uniform definition of response and variable dosage schedules. All histologies were lumped together, and quality control was relatively poor.

An additional problem with these earlier studies as well as current studies to a certain extent was the nature of the patients with advanced or recurrent disease. Virtually all patients had received prior therapy with radiation. This not only rendered evaluation of pelvic disease very difficult but also made response less likely and probably drug delivery to pelvic neoplasm more erratic. Patients furthermore often had ureteral compression and

E.A. Surwit, D.S. Alberts (eds) Cervix Cancer.
 ISBN 0-89838-822-8. Printed in the Netherlands.

resultant renal impairment and hence were less than ideal candidates particularly for such nephrotoxic agents as cisplatin.

Despite these difficulties, efforts to identify active agents have increased in the last decade primarily as a result of the studies of the Gynecologic Oncology Group (GOG). In addition, patients with squamous cell carcinoma which accounts for a large majority of cervix cancer have been studied separately from patients with other histologies. These recent trials have added considerably to knowledge of drug activity and have resulted in the identification of at least one highly active agent in squamous cell carcinomas. The review of these data will be divided into those studies which concern primarily squamous cell carcinoma and those which look at only non-squamous carcinoma.

Squamous cell carcinoma of the cervix

Squamous cell carcinoma of the cervix comprises about 85% of all cancer of the uterine cervix. Data on the use of single agents in this disease derive from two sources: older compiled data perhaps 10–15% of which are cases of non-squamous cervix carcinoma and the more recent GOG studies which include only squamous carcinoma.

Approved cytotoxic agents

Cisplatin

By far the best studied and most active single agent in squamous cell carcinoma of the cervix is cisplatin. Cisplatin (cis-diamminedichloroplatinum II) is a platinum coordination complex in which the two chlorides reside in the cis position and the platinum valence is 2. The principle mechanism of action is thought to be activation in a low chloride environment to a bifunctional alkylating agent as a result of the two chloride ions leaving the molecule [3], although other mechanisms have been proposed [4].

Adverse effects associated with cisplatin are numerous and include among others: nephrotoxicity, peripheral neuropathy, ototoxicity, anaphylactic reactions, and myelosuppression [5]. Of particular importance in the patient with cervix cancer is the nephrotoxicity, which must be taken into account in patients susceptible to obstructive uropathy related to tumor. Vigorous hydration with or without mannitol has been noted to prevent a significant proportion of the reported cases of nephrotoxicity. As a result, more recent trials have noted a cumulative peripheral neuropathy to be of greater significance in limiting the total dose of cisplatin which could be given over time.

The GOG has studied cisplatin in patients with squamous cervix carcinoma extensively (Table 1) [6–8]. The first series consisted of 34 patients [6], 22 of whom had received no prior chemotherapy, treated with 50 mg/m^2 every 3 weeks. Eleven of the 22 with no prior chemotherapy responded (50%), while two of the 12 with prior chemotherapy (17%) demonstrated regression of disease. These data suggested a high order of activity.

Based on initial results, the GOG undertook a larger trial in previously untreated patients comparing the initial regimen with two higher dose schedules, 100 mg/m^2 as a single dose every 3 weeks and 20 mg/m^2 daily times five every 3 weeks [7]. A total of 440 patients were randomized to one of the tree regimens. Although the study failed to identify an initial goal of a 15% difference in response, the observed 10% advantage for the 100 mg/m^2 regimen was significantly better than the 50 mg/m^2 schedule ($p = 0.05$). There was, however, no difference in progression-free interval or survival; and the clinical significance of a 10% difference in response was considered problematic.

The third GOG trial of single-agent cisplatin, also in patients with no prior chemotherapy, compared the 50 mg/m^2 regimen given as a 1 mg/min infusion to the same dose given over a longer period of 24 h with the dual goal of seeking less nausea and vomiting and better response [8]. There was no observed advantage for the prolonged infusion in regard to response, but a significantly greater number of pattents receiving the 24 hour infusion experienced no nausea and vomiting.

This series of three trials confirms two significant facts. First, cisplatin is clearly active against squamous cell carcinoma. The overall response rate of 23%, although not as high as the initial report of a response rate of 50%, appears firm and is higher than that reported for any other single agent. Secondly, modification of the original 50 mg/m^2 dose and schedule does not

Table 1. GOG studies of cisplatin as a single agent in squamous cell carcinoma of the cervix.

Regimen	Patients	Response (%)
GOG 26C [6]		
50mg/m^2 Q 3 weeks	34	13 (38%)
GOG 43 [7]		
50 mg/m^2 Q 3 weeks	150	31 (21%)
100 mg/m^2 Q 3 weeks	166	52 (31%)
20 mg/m^2 × 5 days Q 3 weeks	128	32 (25%)
GOG 64 [8]		
50 mg/m^2 Q 3 weeks bolus	156	23 (15%)
50 mg/m^2 Q 3 weeks CI*	148	27 (18%)
Total	782	178 (23%)

* Continuous infusion.

offer any identifiable advantage in terms of increased response rate or improved survival.

Experience with singe agent cisplatin outside of the Gynecologic Oncology Group is limited (Table 2) [9–11]. A total of only 33 patients serves to confirm that cisplatin has activity but allows for no conclusions about level of efficacy. The GOG data, however, include sufficient patients to render observations of activity firm beyond reasonable question.

Alkylating agents

Those drugs classified as alkylating agents are highly reactive compounds which act to substitute alkyl groups for hydrogen atoms of macromolecules such as nucleic acids [12]. These substitutions lead to breaks and cross-links in DNA strands and thus to interference with the functioning of DNA molecules. Major adverse effects of these agents include: myelosuppression, nausea and vomiting, alopecia, and a risk for second malignancies as well as adverse effect specific to each compound.

Table 2. Non-GOG trials of cisplatin in squamous cell carcinoma of the uterine cervix.

Regimen				Patients	Responses (%)	Reference
Treated						
120 mg/m^2	Q	3–4	weeks	11	5 (45%)	9
75 mg/m^2	Q	3	weeks	4	0 (0%)	10
5 mg/m^2 × 5 days	Q	3–4	weeks	1	1 (100%)	10
0.75 mg/kg	Q	4–6	weeks	2	0 (0%)	10
Total				18	6 (33%)	
Untreated						
75 mg/m^2	Q	3	weeks	4	0 (0%)	10
3 mg/kg	Q	3	weeks	3	3 (100%)	10
50 mg/m^2	Q	3	weeks	8	3 (38%)	11
Total				15	6 (40%)	

Table 3. Alkylating agents in patients with carcinoma of the cervix.

Drug	Patients	Responses (%)	References
Nitrogen mustard derivatives			
Cyclophosphamide	251	38 (15%)	13, 14
Chlorambucil	44	11 (25%)	13, 15
Melphalan	20	4 (20%)	13
Nitrosoureas			
Methyl CCNU	94	7 (7%)	13, 16
CCNU	63	3 (5%)	13, 16

Two of the five major classes of alkylating agents, the nitrogen mustard derivatives and the nitrosoureas, have been evaluated in cervix carcinoma (Table 3). These data for the most part represent older, compiled data and hence include a small proportion of non-squamous carcinoma. Among the nitrogen mustard derivatives, the best studied agent is cyclophosphamide [13, 14] with a modest response rate of 15% in 251 patients treated. The only other members of this class evaluated in more than ten patients include chlorambucil [13, 15] and melphalan [13]. Both agents appear to have moderate activity in a relatively small number of patients compiled from several series.

Two nitrosoureas, CCNU and methyl CCNU, have been evaluated in a relatively large number of patients [13, 16]. Of the 63 patients receiving CCNU, 58 were a part of a single trial by the GOG in which only two responses were observed [16]. Similarly, 62 of the 94 patients receiving methyl CCNU were a part of the same GOG study with only three responses [16]. These data suggest minimal, insignificant activity for the nitrosoureas.

Antibiotics

Three approved antitumor antibiotics have been evaluated in cervix carcinoma. Most of these data are derived from earlier compiled series fraught with all the problems of such information [17].

Bleomycin is actually a collection of 13 different polypeptides [18]. The drug acts to cause scission of both single-stranded and double-stranded DNA with its major effect occurring in G2 and M phases of the cell cycle. Adverse effects include anaphylactic reactions, fever with or without sweating and dehydration associated with hypotension, skin and mucous membrane reactions, alopecia, and both acute and delayed pulmonary toxicity [19]. The most significant of these is the delayed lung damage which increases in likelihood with increasing total dose of drug [20]. From collected data from multiple series [17], 172 patients were identified as having received bleomycin as a single agent for squamous cell carcinoma of the cervix. Seventeen (10%) were responders. These data suggest that the drug has minimal activity against squamous cell carcinoma of the uterine cervix.

Mitomycin is an antibiotic composed of three potentially active groups: quinone, urethane, and aziridine moieties. *In vivo*, the drug is activated to an alkylating agent principally by reduction of the quinone group [21]. Primary activity is directed at DNA. Adverse effects include myelosuppression, nausea and vomiting, nephrotoxicity, alopecia, severe tissue necrosis at sites of extravasation, interstitial pneumonitis, and possible cardiotoxicity [21]. The most significant toxicity is the cumulative, profound, and prolonged myelosuppression affecting all three formed elements. In addition,

Table 4. Antitumor antibiotics as single agents in patients with squamous cell carcinoma of the cervix.

Drug	Patients	Responses (%)	References
Doxorubicin	205	33 (16%)	17, 25–30
Bleomycin	172	17 (10%)	17
Mitomycin-C	18	4 (22%)	17

nadir counts occur at a longer interval of 3 to 8 weeks after drug administration. Only 18 patients with squamous cell carcinoma of the cervix have been reported as having received the drug as a single agent [17]. Four (22%) were noted to respond. These data suggest possible moderate activity for the drug.

Doxorubicin is the only approved member of the anthracycline family to have been used in a significant number of patients with cervix carcinoma. This drug is a hydroxylated congener of daunorubicin which appears to act by intercalating between adjoining nucleotide pairs of the DNA helix structure [22]. Adverse effects include myelosuppression, cardiotoxicity, severe local tissue necrosis at sites of extravasation, alopecia, radiosensitization, stomatitis, nausea and vomiting, diarrhea, and hyperpigmentation of skin [23]. Although acute myelosuppression is often the dose-limiting toxicity, cardiotoxocity is the most significant adverse effect. Cardiotoxicity [24] may occur as acute effects (pericarditis/myocarditis and acute arrhythmias such as premature atrial and ventricular contractions and supraventricular tachyarrhytmias) or as more serious delayed effects such as intractable congestive heart failure. The frequency of congestive failure is related to total dose and increases significantly at cumulative doses exceeding 550 mg/m^2. Doxorubicin has been tested as a single agent in a total of 205 patients with carcinoma of the cervix [17, 25–30]. Thirty-three (16%) of these patients responded objectively to therapy. This frequency of response is reasonably consistent through the various series and hence seems firm. These data suggest that doxorubicin has moderate activity against squamous cell carcinoma of the cervix.

Antimetabolites

The antimetabolites are a heterogeneous group of compounds that act as false substrates for biochemical processes and hence interfere with vital metabolic steps within a cell. The major focus of activity is the S phase of the cell cycle, and the principal mechanism of action is the interference with synthesis of DNA and possibly other macromolecules. This group includes three major types of substances: folate antagonists, purine antagonists, and pyrimidine antagonists. Three approved antimetabolites have been eva-

Table 5. Antimetabolites as single agents in patients with squamous cell carcinoma of the cervix.

Drug	Patients	Responses (%)	References
5-Fluorouracil	142	29 (20%)	17, 32
Methotrexate	96	17 (18%)	17, 25
6-Mercaptopurine	18	1 (5%)	17

luated as single agents in patients with carcinoma of the cervix, one from each of the three classses (Table 5) [13].

The only approved folate antagonist evaluated in carcinoma of the cervix is methotrexate [17, 25]. This agent acts by binding to dihydrofolate reductase thereby to block the reduction of dihydrofolate to tetrafolate. This inhibits synthesis of thymidylic acid and also purines [31]. Adverse effects include principally myelosuppression, nausea and vomiting, diarrhea, mucositis, a variety of dermatologic effects, hepatotoxicity including delayed development of cirrhosis with long-term therapy, and renal failure particularly in those patients receiving high dose therapy. Many of these effects may be ameliorated by the administration of reduced folates (citrovorum factor rescue) thus to enable tolerance of much higher doses of the drug.

Use of methotrexate as a single agent has been reported in 96 patients, 17 (18%) of whom were observed to develop an objective response [17, 25]. Eighty-nine of the 96 received conventional doses of the drug without rescue with citrovorum factor, while seven received high-dose therapy with rescue. Two of the 17 responses were observed in the seven receiving high dose therapy, but there is no indication that this offered greater patient benefit. Methotrexate thus appears to possess moderate activity against carcinoma of the cervix.

The most extensively studied antimetabolite is the pyrimidine antagonist 5-fluorouracil [17, 32]. This drug is a fluorinated pyrimidine which competes for the enzyme thymidylate synthetase and thus prevents the conversion of uracil deoxyribotide to thymidine. This ultimately interferes with DNA synthesis. Adverse effects include myelosuppression, nausea and vomiting, diarrhea, mucositis, alopecia, maculopapular rash, cerebellar abnormalities, and hyperpigmentation over veins through which the drug is administered.

The reported use of 5-fluorouracil as a single agent in carcinoma of the cervix includes 142 patients [17, 32]. Twenty-nine responders were observed for a response rate of 20%. Based on these collected data, the drug appears to have moderate activity in carcinoma of the cervix.

The only purine antagonist to be evaluated in carcinoma of the cervix is 6-mercaptopurine in the relatively small number of 18 patients [17]. Only one responder (5%) was observed. This agent therefore appears to have insignificant activity in this disease.

Plant alkaloids

The periwinkle plant and the May-apple plant have provided three currently approved alkaloids that have been evaluated in patients with carcinoma of the cervix. All three of these compounds act primarily in M phase of the cell cycle to interfere with the formation of the mitotic spindle and result in a metaphase arrest [33, 34].

The two alkaloids isolated from the periwinkle plant are vincristine and vinblastine. While both are similar with regard to chemical structure and mechanism of action, the spectum of adverse effects associated with each is different. For vincristine, the major dose-limiting toxicity is neurotoxicity manifested by a peripheral neuropathy with paresthesias and loss of deep-tendon reflexes progressing to severe weakness and by cranial and autonomic neuropathies. For vinblastine, myelosuppression is the major dose-limiting effect. Both drugs will produce local necrosis upon extravasation and alopecia.

The two vinca alkaloids have both been tested as single agents in recent phase II trials in squamous cell carcinoma of the cervix (Table 6). Vincristine [35, 36] was given both as a weekly bolus and as a continuous infusion with no apparent difference by method of administration. Of 55 patients treated, ten were observed to respond (18%). Vinblastine [37] was given as a continuous infusion over 5 days to 20 patients with an observed two objective responses (10%). Both drugs thus appear to have modest activity against squamous cell carcinoma of the cervix.

The podophyllotoxin VP-16-213 (Etoposide) is the only approved podophyllotoxin. Its spectrum of adverse effects is similar to that noted for vinblastine with the major dose-limiting toxicity being myelosuppression. Also noted are nausea, vomiting, diarrhea, alopecia, phlebitis at the injection site, and hypotension upon rapid administration. The drug has been evaluated by the GOG in a series of 31 patients with squamous cell carcinoma of the cervix (Table 6) [38]. There were no observed responses, This agent thus appears to have no appreciable activity in this disease.

Table 6. Plant akaloids as single agents in patients with suqamous cell carcinoma of the cervix.

Drug	Patients	Responses (%)	References
Vincristine	55	10 (18%)	35, 36
Vinblastine	20	2 (10%)	37
VP-16-213	31	0 (0%)	38

Other agents

The only other approved drug with meaningful evaluation in carcinoma of the cervix is the ribonucleotide reductase inhibitor hydroxyurea. This agent is of particular interest because of two reports from the GOG concerning definite benefit associated with the use of the drug concomitantly with radiotherapy in patients with locally advanced carcinoma of the cervix [39, 40]. The drug has been studied in patients with disseminated or recurrent carcinoma of the cervix in only 14 patients with no observed responses [15]. As a single cytotoxic agent, therefore, it appears to have no appreciable activity. Its efficacy in earlier disease is thought to be a result of action as a radiosensitizer.

Investigational cytotoxic agents

Platinum analogues

The significant activity of cisplatin and its rather marked adverse effects have combined to incite interest in the development of analogues which improve on the therapeutic/toxic ratio. A number of these analogues has been developed [41, 43]. The two analogues of greatest current interest in carcinoma of the cervix are cis-diammine-1,1-cyclobutane dicarboxylate platinum II (carboplatin, CBDCA, JM8, NSC 241240) and cis-dichloro-trans-dihydroxy-bis-(isopropylamine)-platinum IV (CHIP, NSC 256927). Phase I trials [44, 45] indicate that the spectrum of adverse effects with these two analogues is markedly different from cisplatin. Myelosuppression appears to be the dose-limiting toxicity for each; while the incidence of neurotoxicity, nephrotoxicity, and gastrointestinal toxicity is greatly reduced.

The GOG is currently conducting a randomized trial of these agents in patients with squamous cell carcinoma of the cervix who had received no prior chemotherapy. The initial phase II experience with each drug from this trial has been reported (Table 8) [46, 47]. Carboplatin yielded six responses in 29 patients (21 %), while CHIP produced five responses among 22 patients (23%). These response rates are quite similar to the overall response rate noted by the GOG in 782 patients treated with cisplatin, and

Table 7. Other approved drugs evaluated as single agents in patients with squamous cell carcinoma of the cervix.

Drug	Patients	Responses (%)	References
Hydroxurea	14	0 (0%)	15

the adverse effects observed in the phase II experiences with the two analogues are comparable to those reported in the phase I trials. Acquisition of a larger experience is in progress as noted. These early results, however, suggest that both analogues are of interest as possible alternatives to cisplatin and deserve further study.

Other investigational agents

In addition to the platinum analogues, 14 other investigational agents have been evaluated in patients with squamous cell carcinoma of the cervix over the last 10 years (Table 9). Ten of these agents were a part of a concerted effort, still on-going, by the GOG to evaluate a number of new agents in squamous cell carcinoma of the cervix [49–57, 60]. Seven of the drugs exhibited little or no activity: AMSA [48, 49], maytansine [54], mitoxantrone [55], PALA [56], piperazinedione [57], spirogermanium [58], and

Table 8. The results of the phase II trials of the GOG using two platinum analogues in patients with squamous cell carcinoma of the cervix. All patients had received no prior chemotherapy.

Drug		Patients	Responses (%)	References
Carboplatin 400 mg/m^2	Q 4 weeks	29	6 (21%)	46
CHIP 300 mg/m^2	Q 4 weeks	22	5 (23%)	47

Table 9. Single agent activity of investigational drugs in patients with squamous cell carcinoma of the cervix.

Drug	Prior Rx	No. of Patients	Responses (%)	References
AMSA	yes	20	0 (0%)	48
	yes	25	1 (4%)	49
Baker's Antifol	yes	32	5 (16%)	50
Dianhydrogalactitol	no	36	7 (19%)	51
Dibromodulcitol	no	47	7 (15%)	52
Hemamethylmelamine	no	64	12 (19%)	17, 30
ICFR-159	yes	28	5 (18%)	53
Maytansine	yes	29	1 (3%)	54
Mitoxantrone	yes	25	2 (8%)	55
PALA	yes	33	0 (0%)	56
Piperazinedione	no	43	2 (5%)	57
Porfiromycin	no	78	17 (22%)	17
Spirogermanium	yes	14	9 (0%)	58
Vindesine	mixed	21	5 (24%)	59
Yoshi 864	yes	18	0 (0%)	60

Yoshi 864 [60]. In each instance of a negative result, all study patients had received prior chemotherapy except for the trial of piperazinedione. The remaining seven drugs appeared to have moderate activity and will be discussed in more detail.

Baker's Antifol (BAF, Triazinate, NSC-139105) is one of a number of inhibitiors of dihydrofolate reductase synthesized by Dr B.R. Baker. This compound, while acting by a mechanism similar to that of methotrexate, differs in that it enters the cell through a different active transport system and hence may have a different spectrum of activity [61]. Adverse effects of Baker's Antifol are similar to those seen with methotrexate except that myelosuppression is somewhat less prominent and the mucosal and dermatologic effects somewhat more marked. The GOG trial [50] employed a weekly schedule (Table 10) in 32 patients previously treated with cisplatin and noted a response in five patients (16 %). This suggests moderate activity similar to that seen with methotrexate with no discernible advantage for the new compound.

Dianhydrogalactitol (Galactitol, DAG, NSC-132313) is the alkali conversion product of dibromodulcitol which is thought to act as an alkylating agent by cross-linking strands of DNA [62]. The only apparent major adverse effect is myelosuppression. A weekly schedule (Table 10) of the drug was studied by the GOG in 36 patients who had squamous cell carcinoma of the cervix and had received no prior chemotherapy [51]. Seven (19 %) of these were observed to respond. These data suggest moderate activity for the drug.

Dibromodulcitol (DBD, NSC-104800), the parent compound for dianhydrogalactitol, appears to act in a similar fashion as an alkylating agent [63]. As in the case of dianhydrogalactitol, the only major adverse effect appears to be myelosuppression. Collaborating Mexican and U.S. investigators studied 47 previously untreated patients with a daily times 10 schedule (Table 10) with a total of seven observed responses [52]. All seven responders were

Table 10. Representative dose and schedule of investigational agents with apparent moderate activity against squamous cell carcinoma of the cervix.

Drug	Dose and schedule	References
Baker's Antifol	500 mg/m^2 IV weekly	50
Dianhydrogalactitol	60 mg/m^2 IV weekly	51
Dibromodulcitol	180–240 mg/m^2 IV × 10 days	52
Hexamethylmelamine	12 mg/kg/day × 21 days Q 7 weeks	17, 30
ICRF-159	2.5 gm/m^2 IV weekly	53
Porfiromycin	7.5–10.5 mg/m^2 twice weekly × 6	17
Vindesine	3 mg/m^2 IV weekly × 6	59

seen among the 29 Mexican patients treated (24%), whereas none of the 18 U.S. patients responded. The explanation for this disparity was not clear. While the agent would appear to have moderate activity in squamous cell carcinoma of the cervix, the disparity of results between the two teams of investigators requires that the activity be confirmed in additional trials.

Hexamethylmelamine (HMM, NSC-13875) is a melamine derivative of cyanuric chloride structurally similar to the alkylating agent triethylenemelamine (TEM), but its exact mechanism of action is not clear [64]. Some evidence suggests that the drug is not cross-resistant with standard alkylating agents [65, 66]. The myelosuppressive effects of hexamethylmelamine are mild and not dose-limiting. Of greater significance are the gastrointestinal toxicity (anorexia, nausea, vomiting, diarrhea, and abdominal cramps) and the neurotoxicity (both peripheral and central effects). In two separate series [17, 30], a total of 64 previously untreated patients with squamous cell carcinoma of the cervix received the drug (Table 10) with 12 observed responses (19%). These data suggest moderate drug activity.

ICRF-159 (Razoxane, NSC-129143) is a derivative of the chelating agent EDTA [67] which exerts an antitumor effect by a mechanism similar to that of the alkylating agents [68]. Adverse effects include dose-limiting myelosuppression and gastrointestinal toxicity. Alopecia and a papular dermatitis have also been reported. The drug was tested by the GOG in a weekly schedule in a series of 28 previously untreated patients with squamous cell carcinoma of the cervix. Five responses were noted for a response rate of 18%. This suggests that ICRF-159 has moderate activity in the weekly schedule tested.

Porfiromycin is from the same family of compounds as mitomycin [21] with a similar mechanism of action and essentially identical spectrum of adverse effects. Older, compiled data from several series [17] reflect 78 previously untreated patients with carcinoma of the cervix who received porfiromycin as a single agent. There were 17 responses reported for a response rate of 22%. This suggests at least moderate activity for the drug, but the fact that these data are compiled from several series suggests that confirmation of activity should be sought if porfiromycin is to be considered for further use.

Finally, the vinca alkaloid vindesine (DVA, Lilly CT-3231), a plant alkaloid with properties similar to those of vinblastine, was tested in a series of 21 patients by investigators of the EORTC [59]. All patients had squamous cell carcinoma of the cervix. Sixteen had received some prior chemotherapy; among these, four responses were seen. Among the five with no prior chemotherapy, one response was observed. The overall response rate for the weekly schedule (Table 10) was 24%. These data suggest moderate to high activity for vindesine.

Table 11. Single agent activity in trials of the GOG in patients with non-squamous carcinoma of the cervix.

Drug	No. of patients	Responses (%)	References
Piperazinedione	14	2 (14%)	69
Cisplatin	20	4 (20%)	69
VP-16-213	19	1 (5%)	70
Galactitol	27	2 (8%)	71
ICRF-159	25	1 (4%)	72

Non-squamous carcinoma of the cervix

Most studies of chemotherapy in carcinoma of the cervix have made no attempt to separate non-squamous cancers from the squamous cell carcinomas which comprise the great majority of cervix cancer. Over the last 10 years, the GOG has studied these cases as a discrete but heterogeneous group which is comprised mostly of adenocarcinoma of the cervix. While these lesions are uncommon, the GOG has been able to evaluated the activity of five drugs: piperazinedione [69], cisplatin [69], VP-16-213 [70], galactitol [71], and ICRF-159 [72] (Table 11). Only cisplatin appears to have clearcut activity with four responses in a population of 20 patients (20%) using a dose of 50 mg/m^2 every 3 weeks. While there were two responses among 14 patients treated with piperazinedione, the number of patients treated is too small to permit conclusions about the efficacy of the drug. There is evidence that the other three drugs have little or no activity.

Summary

Prior to 1976, studies of chemotherapy in carcinoma of the cervix reflected poor quality data and no effort to distinguish between the common squamous cell carcinoma of the cervix and other forms of cervix carcinoma. Over the 10 years since 1976, concerted efforts have been made to assess single agent activity in particularly squamous cell carcinoma of the cervix. Based on these efforts, several conclusions can be drawn:

1. The most active drug in the treatment of squamous cell carcinoma of the cervix is cisplatin. While higher dose schedules yield a statistically significant 10% improvement in response rate, this gain is not reflected in gains in progression-free interval and survival. Regardless of dose and schedule, the median duration of response ranges from 4–6 months and median survival 6–9 months with cisplatin alone.

2. Platinum analogues require further study but appear to offer an improved therapeutic/toxic ratio with no loss of efficacy.
3. A number of additional drugs appear to have moderate activity in squamous cell carcinoma of the cervix. These include: mustard-type alkylating agents, doxorubicin, mitomycin and porfiromycin, 5-fluorouracil, methotrexate, the vinca alkaloids, hexamethylmelamine, Baker's Antifol, dianhydrogalactitol, dibromodulcitol, and ICRF-159.
4. Drugs tested with insignificant activity include: the nitrosoureas, 6-mercaptopurine, VP-16-213, bleomycin, hydroxyurea, AMSA, maytansine, mitoxantrone, PALA, piperazinedione, spirogermanium, and Yoshi 864.
5. Only five agents have been tested as single agents in patients with non-squamous carcinoma of the cervix, and only cisplatin appears to have significant activity. Those drugs which appear to have insignificant activity include: VP-16-213, dianhydrogalactitol, and ICRF-159. An insufficient number of patients were studied with piperazinedione to allow conclusions to be drawn.

If chemotherapy is to offer patients with advanced or recurrent carcinoma of the cervix substantial benefit in the future, research efforts must be targeted to the identification of highly activity agents other than cisplatin so that reasonable platinum-based combination chemotherapy can be devised and tested. Study patients, if at all possible, should be patients with no prior chemotherapy and good indicator lesions so that drug assessment can be fair and precise. This general research direction has been adopted by the Gynecologic Oncology Group in an effort to improve systemic treatment for these patients.

References

1. Silverberg E, Lubera J. 1986. Cancer statistics, 1986. Ca-A Cancer J Clin 36:9-25.
2. DeVita V, Wasserman T, Young R, Carter S. 1976. Perspectives on research in gynecologic oncology. Cancer 38:509–525.
3. Roberts J, Pascoe J. 1972. Cross-linking of complementary strands of DNA in mammalian cells by antitumor platinum compounds. Nature (Lond) 235:282–284.
4. Rosenberg B. 1975. Possible mechanisms for the antitumor activity of platinum coordination complexes. Cancer Chemother Rep 59:589–598.
5. Rozencweig M *et al.* 1977. Ann Intern Med 86:803.
6. Thigpen T, Shingleton H, Homesley H, Lagasse L, Blessing, J. 1981. Cis-platinum in treatment of advanced or recurrent squamous cell carcinoma of the cervix: a phase II study of the Gynecologic Oncology Group. Cancer 48:899–903.
7. Bonomi P, Blessing J, Stehman F, DiSaia P, Walton L, Major F. 1985. Randomized trial of three cisplatin dose schedules in squamous cell carcinoma of the cervix (a Gynecologic Oncology Group study). J Clin Oncol 3:1079–1085.

8. Thigpen T, Blessing J, DiSaia P, Shingleton H, Fowler W. 1986. Cisplatin in the management of patients with advanced or recurrent squamous carcinoma of the cervix: effects of prolonged infusion. Proc ASCO (in press).
9. Cohen C, Castro-Marin A, Deppe G, Bruckner H, Holland J. 1978. Chemotherapy of advanced recurrent cervical cancer with platinum II - a preliminary report. Proc ASCO 19:401.
10. Baker L. 1980. Cis-platin in treatment of cervical and endometrial cancer patients. In: Cis-platin: Current Status and New Developments (J Prestayko, S Crooke, S Carter, eds). Academic Press, New York, pp 403–409.
11. Baker L, Boutselis J, Alberts D *et al.* 1985. Combination chemotherapy for patients with disseminated carcinoma of the uterine cervix. Proc ASCO 4:120.
12. Ludlum D. 1967. Reaction of nitrogen mustard with synthetic polynucleotides. Biochim Biophys Acta 142:282–284.
13. Muscato M, Perry M, Yarbro J. 1982. Chemotherapy of cervical carcinoma. Sem Oncol 9:373.
14. Omura G, Velez G, birch R. 1981. Phase II randomized study of doxorubicin, vincristine, and 5-FU versus cyclophosphamide in advanced squamous cell carcinoma of the cervix. Cancer Treat Rep 65:901.
15. Thigpen T, Vance R, Balducci L, Blessing J. 1981. Chemotherapy in the management of advanced or recurrent cervical and endometrial carcinoma. Cancer 48:658.
16. Omura G, Shingleton H, Creasman W, Blessing J, Boronow R. 1978. Chemotherapy of advanced gynecologic cancer with nitrosoureas: a randomized trial of CCNU and methyl CCNU in carcinoma of the cervix, corpus, vaginal, valva and tube. Cancer Treat Rep 62:833–835.
17. Wasserman T, Carter S. 1977. The integration of chemotherapy into combined modality treatment of solid tumors: VIII Cervical Cancer. Cancer Treat Rev 4:25–46.
18. Crooke S, Bradner W. 1976. Bleomycin: a review. J Med 7:333–428.
19. Blum R, Carter S, Agre K. 1973. A clinical review of bleomycin — a new, antineoplastic agent. Cancer 31:903–914.
20. Rudders R, Hensley G. 1973. Bleomycin pulmonary toxicity. Chest 63:626–628.
21. Crooke S, Bradner W. 1976. Mitomycin C: a review. Cancer Treat Rev 3:121–139.
22. DiMarco A. 1972. Adriamycin: the therapeutic activity on experimental tumors. In: International Symposium on Adriamycin, (S Carter *et al.*, eds). Springer Verlag, New York, pp 53–63.
23. Blum R, Carter S. 1974. Adriamycin: a new anticancer drug with significant clinical activity. Ann Intern Med 80:249–259.
24. Rinehart J, Lewis R, Balcerzak S. 1974. Adriamycin cardiotoxicity in man. Ann Intern Med 81:475–478.
25. Cavins J, Geisler H. 1978. Treatment of advanced, unresectable, cervical carcinoma already subjected to complete irradiation therapy. Gynecol Oncol 6:256–260.
26. Piver M, Barlow J, Xynos F. 1978. Adriamycin alone or in combination in 100 patients with carcinoma of the cervix or vagina. Am J Obstet Gynecol 131:311–313.
27. Malkasian G, Decker D, Green S, Edmondson J, Jeffries J, Webb M. 1981. Treatment of recurrent and metastatic carcinoma of the cervix: comparison of doxorubicin with a combination of vincristine and 5-fluorouracil. Gynecol Oncol 11:235–239.
28. Greenberg B, Kardinal C, Pajek T, Bateman J. 1977. Adriamycin versus adriamycin and bleomycin in advanced epidermoid carcinoma of the cervix. Cancer Treat Rep 61:1383–1384.
29. Wallace H, Hreshchyshyn M, Wilbanks G, Boronow R, Fowler W, Blessing J. 1978. Comparison of the therapeutic effect of adriamycin alone versus adriamycin plus vincristine versus adriamycin plus cyclophosphamide in the treatment of advanced carcinoma of the cervix. Cancer Treat Rep 62:1435–1441.

30. Freeman R, Herson J, Wharton J, Rutledge F. 1980. Single agent chemotherapy for recurrent carcinoma of the cervix. Cancer Clin Trials 3:345–350.
31. Werkheiser W. 1963. The biochemical, cellular, and pharmacological action and effects of the folic acid antagonists. Cancer Res 23:1277–1285.
32. Malkasian G, Decker D, Jorgensen E. 1977. Chemotherapy of carcinoma of the cervix. Gynecol Oncol 5:109–120.
33. Noble R, Beer C. 1968. Experimental observations concerning the mode of action of vinca alkaloids. In: The Vinca Alkaloids in the Chemotherapy of Malignant Disease, (W Shedden, ed). John Sherratt and Sons, Alburcham, England, pp 4–11.
34. Krishan A, Paikg K, Frei E III. 1975. Cytofluorometric studies on the action of podophyllotoxin and epipodophyllotoxins (VM-26 and VP-16-213) on the cell cycle travers of human lymphoblasts. J Cell Biol 66:521–530.
35. Bonomi P, Yordan E. 1984. Chemotherapy of cervical carcinoma. In: Chemotherapy of Gynecologic Cancer (G Deppe, ed). Alan R. Liss, Inc., New York, pp 103–124.
36. Jobson V, Jackson D, Homesley H *et al.* 1983. Treatment of recurrent gynecologic malignancies with prolonged intravenous vincristine infusion. Proc ASCO 2:149.
37. Kavanagh J, Copeland L, Gershenson D *et al.* 1985. Continuous infusion vinblastine in refractory carcinoma of the cervix: a phase II trial. Gynecol Oncol 21:211.
38. Slayton R, Creasman W, Petty W *et al.* 1979. Phase II trial of VP-16-213 in treatment of advanced squamous cell carcinoma of the cervix and adenocarcinoma of the ovary: a Gynecologic Oncology Group study. Cancer Treat Rep 63:2089.
39. Hreshchyshyn M, Aron B, Boronow R *et al.* 1979. Hydroxyurea or placebo combined with radiation to treat stage IIIB and IV cervical cancer confined to the pelvis. Int J Rad Oncol Biol Phys 5:317.
40. Stehman F, Jobson V, Bundy B, Fowler W, Whitney C. A randomized trial of hydroxyurea vs misonidazole adjunct to radiation therapy in stages IIB, III, IVA carcinoma of the cervix: a Gynecologic Oncology Group study. Gynecol Oncol (in press).
41. Bradner W, Rose W, Huftalen J. 1980. Antitumor activity of platinum analogs. In: Cisplatin: Current Status and New Developments A Prestayko, S Crooke, S Carter, eds). Academic Press, New York, pp. 171–182.
42. Wolpert-DeFilippes M. 1980. Antitumor activity of cisplatin analogs. In: Cisplatin: Current Status and New Developments A Prestayko, S Crooke, S Carter, eds). Academic Press, New York, pp 183–191.
43. Harrap K, Jones M, Wilkinson R, Clink H, Sparrow S, Mitchley B, Clarke S, Veasey A. 1980. Antitumor toxic and biochemical properties of cisplatin and eight other platinum complexes. In: Cisplatin: Current Status and New Developments (A Prestayko, S Crooke, S Carter, eds). Academic Press, New York, pp 193–212.
44. Calvert A, Harland S, Newell D, Siddik Z, Jones A, McElwain T, Raju S, Wiltshaw E, Smith E, Baker J, Peckham M, Harrap K. 1982. Early clinical studies with cis-diammine-1,1-cyclobutane dicarboxylate platinum II. Cancer Chemother Pharmacol9:140–147.
45. Creaven P, Mittleman A, Pendyala L, Tseng M, Pontes E, Spurelding M, Moayeir H, Madejeruiaz S. 1982. Phase I study of a new anti-neoplastic platinum analogue, cis-dichloro-transdihydroxy-bis (isopropyllamine) platinum IV (CHIP). Proc ASCO 1:22.
46. Arseneau J, Hatch K, Stehman F, Blessing J. 1985. Phase II study of carboplatin in advanced squamous cell carcinoma of cervix. Proc ASCO 4:120.
47. McGuire W, Blassing J, Stehman F, Hatch K. 1985. Phase II study of CHIP in advanced squamous cell carcinoma of the cervix. Proc ASCO 4:121.
48. Hilgers R, Legha S, Boutselis J *et al.* 1984. Amsacrine (m-AMSA) in squamous cell carcinoma of the uterine cervix: a Southwest Oncology Group study. Cancer Treat Rep 68:443.

49. Bonomi P, Blessing J, Sedlacek T *et al.* 1983. Phase II trial of AMSA in patients with advanced or recurrent squamous cell carcinoma of the cervix: a Gynecologic Oncology Group study. Cancer Treat Rep 67:197.
50. Arseneau J, Bundy B, Dolan T *et al.* 1982. Phase II study of Baker's Antifol in advanced squamous cell carcinoma of the cervix. Am J Clin Oncol 5:61.
51. Stehman F, Blom J, Blessing J *et al.* 1983. Phase II trial of galactitol 1,2:5,6-Dianhydro (NSC 132313) in the treatment of advanced gynecologic malignancies: a Gynecologic Oncology Group study. Gynecol Oncol 15:381.
52. Lira-Puerto V, Piccart M, Wiernik P *et al.* 1985. A comparison of US and Mexican experience with single drug therapy in advanced cervical cancer (NCI-PAHO and ECOG study). Proc ASCO 4:117.
53. Conroy J, Lewis G, Blessing J *et al.* 1984. ICRF-159 (razoxane) in patients with advanced squamous cell carcinoma of the uterine cervix. Am J Clin Oncol 7:131.
54. Thigpen T, Ehrlich C, Conroy J, Blessing J. 1983. Phase II study of maytansine in the treatment of advanced or recurrent squamous cell carcinoma of the cervixb: a Gynecologic Oncology Group study. Am J Clin Oncol 6:427.
55. Muss H, Sutton G, Bundy B, Hatch K. Mitoxantrone in patients with advanced cervical carcinoma: a phase II study of the Gynecologic Oncology Group. Am J Clin Oncol (in press).
56. Muss H, Bundy B, DiSaia P *et al.* 1984. PALA in advanced carcinoma of the cervix. Am J Clin Oncol 7:741.
57. Thigpen T, Blessing J, Homesley H, Adcock L. 1983. Phase II trial of piperazinedione in the treatment of advanced or recurrent squamous cell carcinoma of the cervix: a Gynecologic Oncology Group study. Am J Clin Oncol 6:423.
58. Brenner F, Forastiere A, Rosenschein N *et al.* 1982. A phase II study of spirogermanium in patients with advanced carcinomas of the ovary and cervix. Proc ASCO 1:115.
59. Vermorken J, Pecorelli S, Mangioni C *et al.* 1984. Phase II study of vindesine in disseminated squamous cell carcinoma of the uterine cervix. Proc ASCO 3:165.
60. Slavik M, Muss H, Blassing J. 1983. Phase II clinical study of Yoshi 864 in squamous cell carcinoma of the uterine cervix. Cancer Treat Rep 67:195.
61. Skeel R, Sawicki W, Cashmore A, Bertino J. 1973. The basis for the disparate sensitivity of L1210 leukemia and Walker 256 carcinoma to a new triazine folate antagonist. Cancer Res 33:2972–2976.
62. Hidvegi E, Lonai P, Holland J *et al.* 1067. The effect of mannitolmyleran and two new dibromohexitols on the metabolic activities of nucleic acids and proteins. J biochem Pharmacol 16:2143–2153.
63. Csanyi E, Halasz M. 1967. Cross-resistance studies on 1,6-dibromodideoxy-D-mannitol (DBM)-resistant Yoshida S.C. Sarcoma. Br J Cancer 21:353–357.
64. Worzalla J *et al.* 1974. Metabolism of hexamethylmelamine-ring-C14 in rats and man. Cancer Res 34:2669–2674.
65. Talita H, Didolkar M. 1974. Effects of hexamethylmelamine on small cell carcinoma of the lung. Cancer Chemother Rep 58:371–374.
66. Wamplu G, Mellette S, Kumperming M, Regelson W. 1972. Hexamethylmelamine in the treatment of advanced cancer. Cancer Chemother Rep 56:505–514.
67. Creighton A, Hellman K, Whitecross S: 1969. Antitumor activity in a series of bisdiketopiperazines. Nature (Lond) 222:384–385.
68. Creighton A, Birnie G. 1970. Biochemical studies on growth-inhibitor bisdioxopiperazines. I. Effect on DNA, RNA and protein synthesis in mouse-embryo fibroblasts. Int J Cancer 5:47–54.
69. Thigpen T, Blessing J, Fowler W *et al.* Phase II trials of cisplatin and piperazinedione as single agents in the treatment of advanced or recurrent non-squamous carcinoma of the cervix: a Gynecologic Oncology Group study. Cancer Treat Rep (in press).

70. Slayton R, Blessing J, Homesley H. 1984. Phase II trial of etoposide in the management of advanced or recurrent non-squamous cell carcinoma of the cervix. Cancer Treat Rep 68:1513.
71. Stehman F, Blessing J, Homesley H *et al.* 1984. Phase evaluation of dianhydrogalactitol in the treatment of advanced non-squamous cervical carcinoma: a Gynecologic Oncology Group study. Invest New Drugs 3:331.
72. Homesley H, Blessing J, Lewis G. J Clin Onc Submitted for publication.

10. Combination chemotherapy of advanced cervix cancer

DEAN E. BRENNER

Introduction

Enormous strides have been made in the use of cytotoxic chemotherapeutic agents. The development, evaluation, and incorporation of these compounds has been the major effort of the clinical oncologist for the last two decades. Combination therapy has been shown to be superior to single agent therapy and has improved the response rates, durations of survival, and quality of life in many, previously hopeless solid tumors, such as advanced testicular, breast, and ovarian carcinomas.

Unfortunately, epidermoid carcinomas as a group, and carcinomas of the cervix in particular, remain among the most difficult tumors to successfully treat with chemotherapy. A defined role for chemotherapy remains to be established for these tumors. Little potential for chemotherapy induced cure has been documented. Today, cytotoxic chemotherapy is generally reserved for patients with resistant, recurrent, or widely metastatic squamous cell tumors.

This chapter will define the difficulties that so many researchers have encountered in treating patients with advanced carcinoma of the cervix, review published reports of multiagent chemotherapy and use this information to suggest future directions of work.

Practical and theoretical difficulties of treating advanced carcinoma of the cervix with systemic chemotherapy

Epidermoid carcinomas

The large majority (90%) of carcinomas of the cervix are of squamous histology [1]. The remainder are adenocarcinomas, adenosquamous carcino-

E.A. Surwit, D.S. Alberts (eds) Cervix Cancer.
 ISBN 0-89838-822-8. Printed in the Netherlands.

mas, and rare cell types [1]. Epidermoid carcinomas have historically been difficult to treat with systemic chemotherapy. These tumors generally have long doubling times. Since most tumor cells will be resting, i.e. not in any phase of the mitotic cycle, they are protected from the effecs of cytotoxic agents [2].

Recent experience in head and neck tumors [3, 4] suggests that squamous tumors can be killed by currently used cytotoxic agents. Emergence of resistant clones is rapid and is associated with a rapid downhill course. Squamous cell tumors of the lung remain one of the most resistant tumors to cytotoxic treatment [5]. Contemporary studies in anal tumors [6] and esophogeal tumors [7] have suggested that multimodality therapy may have an important role in the control of local tumor and possibly locally extensive tumors.

It remains clear that multiagent chemotherapy alone for any of the above listed common squamous cell tumors is not curative. Due to the short response durations in the majority of patients, many investigators have questioned whether the risks of toxicity are worth the benefits of the minimal enhancement of survival associated with standard cytotoxic chemotherapy. From the experience with other squamous tumors that have similar doubling times to that of cervix carcinomas, cytotoxic chemotherapy may have a major role in initial multimodality treatment rather than in a salvage role.

Pelvic scarring due to prior therapy

Since multiagent chemotherapy has been reserved as salvage treatment for patients who have relapsed or persisted after definitive surgical or radiation therapy, or both, pelvic anatomy is distorted. The vascular supply to pelvic tissues and tumor is compromised [8] and fibrosis in the treated pelvis from surgery and radiation therapy is the rule. The tumor is mixed in a diffuse pattern with the fibrosis. If response to chemotherapy is dependent upon local tissue concentrations of drugs, then tumor in the previously treated pelvis will not repond to systemic therapy.

Clinical experience suggests this assertion to be true. A majority of responses to multiagent chemotherapy are found outside the pelvis. Many studies have recounted 'mixed' tumor responses, that is, extrapelvic tumor has responded to treatment while pelvic tumor has progressed.

Efforts to improve local drug delivery [9–12] have met with minimal success. It is possible that the microvasculature is compromised from prior radiation therapy. Therefore, even though high concentrations in the major pelvic vessels are obtained, drug delivery to the tumor remains poor. It is also conceivable that cell clones which have persisted or have been selected for their ability to resist the effects of ionizing irradiation may also be resistant to cytotoxic agents, even at high concentrations.

Poor organ function due to tumor

The anatomic location of cervix carcinomas lends itself to early compromise of key organs. The kidney is primarily affected. Advanced, bulky tumors commonly present with unilateral, sometimes bilateral ureteral obstruction. Renal function is compromised and excretion of toxic compounds and metabolites is delayed. Cisplatin, methotrexate, and bleomycin, all drugs commonly used in carcinoma of the cervix, are primarily excreted through the kidney. Therefore, greater drug-induced toxicity than usual can be expected in patients with cervix carcinoma. Drug doses need modification for systemic toxicity. Such dose reductions will also reduce the amount of drug delivered to the tumor and, ultimately, tumor response.

Organ compromise from prior therapy

Most cervix carcinoma patients have been previously treated with radiation therapy to the pelvis. Radiation portals typically will encompass large bone marrow reserves in the pelvic bones and the humeral heads. Therefore, bone marrow reserves are limited, and relatively low doses of 'nonmyelosuppressive' (e.g. bleomycin) chemotherapy may cause substantial myelosuppression. Dose reductions to accomidate this toxicity compromise drug therapeutic efficacy. If the experience in breast cancer [13] is any guide to therapeutic efficacy, then dose reductions will decrease cervix cancer response rates to chemotherapy as well.

Prior radiation fibrosis and surgical fibrosis may enhance an already partially obstructed ureter. Although surgical or radiation fibrosis alone are uncommon causes of ureteral obstruction [14], prior treatment may well exacerbate the obstruction caused by persistent local tumor, hence reducing renal clearance of chemotherapy.

Problems associated with the design and analysis of multiagent chemotherapy studies of cervix carcinoma

Patient treatment populations

Heterogeneous patient populations make interpretation of most of the nonrandomized studies difficult. Patients may be selected on the basis of measurable disease only. If measurable disease is primarily outside the pelvis, then better treatment results will be observed compared to a study in which the patient population is drawn from patients with pelvic recurrence. Many studies have attempted to control for this variable by analyzing patients according to disease location. While this procedure is helpful it divides the population into segments so small that no useful information can be obtained about treatment efficacy other than determining that extrapelvic tumor responds better than intrapelvic tumor. Some studies have simply excluded all patients with pelvic recurrences. This improves response rates, and perhaps survival rates. Unfortunately, most patients have intrapelvic recurrence.

Defining a response

Earlier multiagent studied did not define a 'response' according to today's standard criteria. Most recent multiagent studies adhere to standard criteria.

Recurrent carcinoma of the cervix is difficult to measure. Since most patients being treated with chemotherapy have undergone surgical and radiation therapy, the pelvis is a fibrotic mass. Unless a clear, obvious lesion is present, such as a crater on the vaginal or cervical surface, which has biopsy proven tumor in it, one cannot be sure that the measured mass is indeed tumor. Hence, data derived solely from physical examination, must be viewed with some suspicion. Disease outside the pelvis is somewhat easier to measure by standard radiologic techniques.

We have expended considerable effort evaluating computed tomography in patients with carcinoma of the cervix confined to the pelvis, both early and late stage [15, 16]. While CT may be able to visualize early, untreated tumor, it does not help distinguish tumor from fibrosis in the late stage patient. It may help define tissue planes for comparison pre and post treatment and may allow some improved measurement of tumor if combined with some type of volume calculation [17]. Still, the definition of a partial response in previously treated pelvic tumors is a major problem affecting the interpretation of treatment results in most published series of multiagent chemotherapy.

The problem of mixed responses

Mixed responses, tumor responses in one anatomic site and progression in another, are common in multiagent chemotherapy studies of cervix carcinoma. Measurable disease in extrapelvic sites such a lung will respond, sometimes completely, while disease in the pelvis progresses. Are mixed responses true responses? Upon comparison of durations of response and survival of patients with true partial responses versus those of nonresponders, patients with mixed responses behaved as nonresponders [46]. Therefore, patients who obtain mixed responses most likely do not gain benefits from treatment and should be coded as nonresponders. In most series, this is indeed the case and most data may not be discarded for inappropriate evaluation of mixed responders.

Dose reductions

Major descrepancies in response and survival among studies from diverse institutions treating patients with identical drug regimens may be the results of differences in the aggressiveness of drug treatment. It is unclear whether clinical dose response relationships exist for cervix carcinoma. Recent experience in a clinical study of cisplatin alone at various doses suggest that higher doses may not enhance response rates over lower, clinically useful doses [18]. The minimum effective dose for cytotoxic agents alone or in combination is unknown.

It is unclear what the effect of dose reductions are upon response and survival data in the treatment of a resistant tumor such as cervix carcinoma. Few of the reviewed studies gave any information as to the frequency or degree of dose reductions. It is conceivable that the same drug combination may provide very different response and survival rates depending upon the dose reduction policies of individual investigators. For example, more aggressive investigations incorporating fewer dose reductions may produce poorer survival results, even in responding patients due to drug induced toxicity. The generally poor physical condition and heavy pretreatment of cervix carcinoma patients coming to multiagent chemotherapy predicts a high rate of severe toxicity and early death.

Study endpoints: response versus survival

What are the appropriate criteria with which to compare studies? Should the 'bottom line' of treatment effectiveness be response rate or survival? This problem has plagued the analysis of solid tumor treatment data for a long time. In the review of multiagent regimens below, I have listed both. Survival must be considered a 'bottom line' figure by which to evaluate the therapeutic efficacy of treatment. If a response can lead to improved survival, so much the better. However, in the case of cervix carcinoma, this is all to often not the case. Partial responses, in particular, should be looked upon with suspicion. Durations of partial responses are short, usually no more than 6 months. In many series, survival in these patients are not improved over nonresponders. Variables such as measurement errors may play an important part in the definition of partial responses, particularly those responses occurring in the pelvis. It is conceivable that the toxicity from the chemotherapy may obviate any benefits accrued from a partial response.

Rationale for multiagent chemotherapy

In 1943, Luria and Delbruck noted that *E. Coli* developed resistance to bacteriophage by expanding clones of bacteria that had spontaneously mutated to a type inherently resistant to infection [19]. Goldie and Coldman [20] applied this principle to the development of resistance by cancer cells to anticancer drugs. Most human cancers have mutation rates in the range of 10^{-6} or higher. The likelihood of having at least one resistant cell line present in a measurable tumor mass (at least 10^7 cells) to a given cytotoxic agent is high. It is less likely that that cells will have *de novo* resistance to multiple cytotoxic agents. Therefore, it is reasonable to attempt treatment of tumor masses with more than one agent in hopes of reducing the number of resistant cells present while improving cell kill.

Skipper *et al.* [21] demonstrated synergistic therapeutic effect of two antineoplastic mechanisms, e.g. an alkylating agent and an antimetabolite. Combining drugs with different mechanisms of action and overlapping toxicity have the following advantages: (1) they provide maximal cell kill within the range of toxicity tolerated by the host for each drug, (2) they can cover a large number of resistant cell clones within a tumor mass, and (3) they can prevent or slow the development of resistant tumor cell lines [22].

It is useful to combine drugs that have single-agent complete response rates rather than partial response rates [22]. Combining drugs with lower response rates will, in most instances, result in less effective therapy.

Single agents active in carcinoma of the cervix

The following agents have activity in carcinoma of the cervix as demonstrated in phase II single agent studies: cyclophosphamide, 5-fluorouracil, methotrexate, vincristine, bleomycin, adriamycin, mitomycin-C, and cisplatin [8, 23, 24]. With the exception of cisplatin, response rates are in the range of 10–25%. Response rates of cisplatin have been reported as high as 50% [25], although recent GOG data suggest a much lower (25%) response rate [18]. Few, if any, complete responses are reported. Response durations are short, 6 months or less, as are survivals in most patients. It is not clear that single agent chemotherapy provides any survival benefit over no treatment, although no studies to date have addressed this question.

Review of combination regimens

Combination chemotherapy regimens for carcinoma of the cervix have been built around three drugs with known activity-adriamycin, bleomycin, and cisplatin. I have arbitrarily divided combination studies into adriamycin, bleomycin, and cisplatin based regimens. Older studies concentrated on adriamycin and bleomycin combinations. New york, since 1980, has primarily concentrated on the use of cisplatin in combination.

Adriamycin-methotrexate

Early studies by Guthrie and Way [26] found the combination of adriamycin (50 mg/m^2) and methotrexate (20 mg/m^2) to induce a high response rate in a small group of patients. The toxicity was substantial, mostly involving mucous membranes. Inadequate data were presented to determine the extent of myelosuppression. When doses were reduced by other investigators [28, 29] response rates dropped precipitously. Most of the adriamycin-methotrexate studies listed in Table 1 reported drug induced deaths from sepsis and bleeding. The high incidence of toxicity could be related to the inexperience of the investigators using a nephrotoxic drug (methotrexate) in a group of patients with compromised renal function. Patient selection in the early studies may play a role in the high response rates. Many of the reported responses were extrapelvic [26, 28, 29, 31]. It is possible, in these early studies, that some authors reported mixed responses as reponses. This may account for the poor durations of response and poor survivals.

The short durations of response and survival do not appear to improve upon the results obtained from adriamycin given alone. Despite the large amount of literature devoted to this combination, no randomized studies of adriamycin alone and the combination with methotrexate have been published. The toxicity and poor treatment results from this combination do not recommend its use as contemporary therapy for advanced carcinoma of the cervix.

Adriamycin in combination with cyclophosphamide, vincristine, or 5-fluorouracil

Cyclophosphamide, vincristine, and 5-fluorouracil all have some activity, albeit minimal, in carcinoma of the cervix and are, therefore, logical candi-

Table 1. Adriamycin and methotrexate in carcinoma of the cervix.

Combination	Evaluable patients	CR	PR	Response (%)	Duration of response (median-months)	Survival (months)	Comments	Author (ref no.)
ADR+MTX	9	6	2	89	NA	4.8	First study, 2 toxic deaths	Guthrie [26]
ADR+MTX	59	12	26	64	NA	14	Varied dosing interval of MTX	Guthrie [27]
ADR+MTX	16	0	2	13	3.3	NA	Lower dose than Guthrie	Haid [28]
ADR+MTX	24	0	7	29	NA	NA	Extrapelvic responders	Papavasiliou [29]
ADR+MTX	15	0	0	0	NA	NA	Not better than ADR alone	Piver [30]
ADR+MTX	24	0	5	21	5	10	Too toxic, no better than ADR alone	Trope [31]
ADR+MTX	22	2	3	23	8	NA	Only isolated lung mets gained benefit	Maillot [32]

ADR = adriamycin; MTX = methotrexate; CR = complete response; PR = partial response.

Table 2. Adriamycin, cyclophosphamide, ± vincristine, ± 5-fluorouracil in carcinoma of the cervix.

Combination	Evaluable patients	CR	PR	Response (%)	Duration of response (median-months)	Survival (months)	Comments	Author (ref no.)
ADR+CTX	10	0	1	10	12	NA	Not useful	Alberts [33]
ADR+CTX	20	1	5	30	4	6	No better than ADR alone	Hanjani [34]
ADR	61	7	5	20	3.3	5.9	Randomized GOG study,	Wallace [35]
ADR+CTX	61	1	8	15	3.4	5.5	all regimens dissap-	
ARD+VCR	52	3	4	13	3.9	7.3	pointing due to short durations of response & survival	
ADR+CTX+VCR	15	1	1	13	NA	5.5	Not useful	Sorbe [36]
ADR+CTX+5FU	36	1	5	17	3–18	8.5	Too toxic, minimal benefit	Piver [37]
ADR+CTX+VCR+5FU	31	1	2	10	NA	7.6	GOG randomized study,	Omura [38]
CTX	30	0	2	7	NA	6.5	disappointing study	

ADR = adriamycin; CTX = cyclophosphamide; VCR = vincristine; 5FU = 5-fluorouracil; CR = complete response; PR = partial response.

dates for combination therapy with adriamycin. Doses of adriamycin in the reviewed combination studies ranged from 40 to 60 mg/m^2, cyclophosphamide from 200 to 500 mg/m^2, and 5-fluorouracil, 500 mg/m^2. The results of these studies are listed in Table 2.

Of most interest is the Gynecologic Oncology Group (GOG) study of Wallace *et al.* [35]. This study is important because of the randomization of the combination against single drug treatment. These data suggest no advantage of the combination over single agent treatment. Furthermore, the combinations were associated with much more toxicity. The doses of adriamycin alone and in combination were comparable. While it is unknown what the degree of dose reduction was among the different institutions of the GOG, the data from the multiinstitutional trial are similar to those from other, single arm, single institutional trials. Another randomized trial of the GOG [38], this one comparing multiagent therapy to cyclophosphamide alone, is remarkable for the lack of difference in response and survival between the two treatment arms. The short durations of response and survival again suggest that these combinations do no improve upon single agent treatment and are not useful for contemporary treatment of advanced cervix carcinoma.

Miscellaneous combination studies with adriamycin

Table 3 reviews miscellaneous studies of adriamycin and methotrexate combinations. Despite the use of different drugs and different doses of the same drugs (e.g. high dose and low dose methotrexate in the studies of Hakes *et al.* [41] and Morrow *et al.* [42] respectively), the response rates are remarkably similar. The study of Day *et al.* [39] with methyl-CCNU and adriamycin draws attention due to a higher than usual response rate. Unfortunately, patients with pelvic tumor only were excluded from entry, thus eliminating a large group of patients who would do poorly with chemotherapy. Despite these special selection criteria, the duration of response and survival in this study are no better than those of adriamycin alone.

Adriamycin and bleomycin

Bleomycin is an ideal drug to test in squamous cell tumors because bleomycin inactivating enzymes are not present in epithelial cells [43]. In early studies listed in Table 4, bleomycin was administered by weekly bolus at a dose of approximately 10 U/m^2. The adriamycin dose varied among the studies from 50 mg/m^2 to an escalation to 90 mg/m^2 given in equal doses over 3 days. The regimens were generally well tolerated with few septic deaths; but there was a constant incidence of pulmonary toxicity.

Table 3. Miscellaneous early combination regimens for advanced cervic carcinoma.

Combination	Evaluable patients	CR	PR	Response (%)	Duration of response (median-months)	Survival (months)	Comments	Author (ref no.)
ADR + MeCCNU	31	9	5	45	4	9.2	Excluded tumor in pelvis only, CRs improved survival	Day [39]
ADR	20	0	4	5	2.5	10	No differences between the arms	Malkasian [40]
VCR + 5FU	21	0	1	21	2.5	6		
VCR + HDMTX	29	0	5	17	4.6	NA	No improvement over low dose MTX	Hakes [41]
VCR + MTX + hydrea	13	0	1	8	NA	3+	Early study, poor results	Morrow [42]

ADR = adriamycin; MeCCNU = methyl CCNU; VCR = vincristine; 5FU = 5-fluoruracil; HDMTX = high dose methotrexate; MTX = methotrexate; hydrea = hydroxyurea; CR = complete response; PR = partial response.

Table 4. Adriamycin + bleomycin for advanced cervix carcinoma.

Combination	Evaluable patients	CR	PR	Response (%)	Duration of response (median-months)	Survival (months)	Comments	Author (ref no.)
ADR+BLEO	8	0	5	63	3	NA		De Paulo [44]
CTX+VCR	11	0	4	36	1.5	NA		
BLEO → ADR	7	1	1	25	3.2	9+, 5	Sequence vs. combinations, no difference between arms	Barlow [45]
ADR+BLEO	15	1	1	13	3.2	6+, 5		
ADR	9	0	5	56	NA	4.5	No difference between arms	Greenberg [46]
ADR+BLEO	11	0	0	0	NA	4.5		
ADR+BLEO	16	0	1	6	NA	NA	Not useful	Piver [30]

ADR = adriamycin; BLEO = bleomycin; CTX = cyclophosphamide; VCR = vincristine.

The studies of Barlow *et al.* [45] and Greenberg *et al.* [46] randomized the combination against bleomycin or adriamycin respectively. The combination was no better than either single agent. Greenberg *et al.* [46] reported mixed responses which they called partial responses. These responses today would not be considered partial responses. The survival data of Barlow *et al.* [45] may not be interpreted because all failures were crossed over to the other treatment arm. The study of Piver *et al.* [30] deserves mention only for its complexity. This work is a published compendium of Piver *et al.*'s sequential clinical studies. Only response rates are given, no duration of response or survival data are available. Since the patient numbers are small in all the treated arms except adriamycin alone (50 patients treated), it is impossible to compare the data and make any conclusions from it. Overall, the response, response duration, and survival data for the combination does not show any improvement over either drug alone.

Bleomycin combinations

Bleomycin-mitomycin C

Based upon the cell kinetic studies *in vitro* [47, 48] Miyamoto *et al.* [49] designed a sequential treatment regimen employing bleomycin, 5 mg daily by continuous infusion for 7 days followed by mitomycin-C, 10 mg. The cycle was to be repeated every 2 weeks. The regimen was devised as a method to sequence the cells to the G2 phase of the mitotic cycle [48, 50]. Mitomycin-C is thought to be most active at the G2-M interface [51]. The long infusion time was used in an attempt to capture more cells in the G2 phase due to the long doubling time of squamous cells [47–51].

Miyamoto *et al.* [49] reported outstanding results with high complete response rates. Unfortunately, the median response duration was short, although some patients had prolonged survivals. In a follow-up study of 63 patients, Miyamoto *et al.* [52] used carboquone as maintenance therapy. The result was heavy toxicity and a reduction in response rate.

These data stimulated a large group of studies from around the world (Table 5) which used the identical regimen. The treatment results did not match those of Miyamoto's, with most response durations and survivals similar to previous multiagent studies.

The descrepancies in response rates and survivals among different groups using the same treatment regimen may be explained with subtle differences in patient selection and in dose reduction schedules. Leichman *et al.* [55] reported mild toxicity and a low response rate of 16% despite higher doses of prior radiation therapy than Miyamoto *et al.* Trope *et al.* [59] reported heavy toxicity with a higher response rate, 36%. Trope *et al.* had a distribution of complete responses and partial responses more comparable to Miyamoto than the other reviewed studies.

Table 5. Bleomycin + mitomycin-C in advanced cervix carcinoma.

Combination	Evaluable patients	CR	PR	Response (%)	Duration of response (median-months)	Survival (months)	Comments	Author (ref no.)
BLEO+MMC	15	12	2	93	4.5	3–30	High response incl. pelvis	Miyamoto [51]
BLEO+MMC	63	39	6	71	4.5	NA	Carboquone for maintenance, heavy toxicity	Miyamoto [52]
BLEO+MMC	4	2	0	50	NA	NA	Too few patients	Llorens [53]
BLEO+MMC	20	1	7	40	2–10	7	Large tumor bulk	Krebs [54]
BLEO+MMC	19	1	2	16	2.5–6	NA	Mild toxicity, more prior RT than Miyamoto	Leichman [55]
BLEO+MMC	23	2	4	26	NA	8+	Selected lower pelvic tumor burden	Boice [56]
BLEO+MMC	9	2	0	22	3.5	NA	Non-irradiated tumor responded	Petrilli [57]
BLEO+MMC	18	0	4	22	3.4	8.5	Regimen of limited use	Greenberg [58]
BLEO+MMC	33	5	7	36	6–12	10	Highly toxic, limited usefullness, some activity	Trope [59]
BLEO+MMC	11	0	1	9	2	NA		Copas [60]

BLEO = bleomycin; MMC = mitomycin-C; CR = complete response; PR = partial response.

Table 6. Multiagent regimens including bleomycin in advanced cervix carcinoma.

Combination	Evaluable patients	CR	PR	Response (%)	Duration of response (median-months)	Survival (months)	Comments	Author (ref no.)
BLEO+MMC+VCR	27	2	11	48	4	NA	Pilot study, thought useful extrepelvic responses	Baker [61]
BLEO+MMC+VCR	50	8	22	60	8.9	5.3	VCR 2×/wk×12 wk,	Baker [62]
BLEO+MMC+VCR	41	6	10	39	16.5	6	BLEO 2×/wk,	
BLEO+MMC+VCR	24	1	5	25	11.9	4.3	BLEO by infusion, VCR 2×/wk less toxic, VCR 1×/wk, BLEO 1×/wk	
BLEO+VCR+MTX	17	1	8	53	2	8	Select pts to evaluate for response	Behnam [63]
BLEO+VCR+MTX	14	0	2	14	2	9	Not useful therapy	Hannigan [64]
BLEO+VCR+MMC	3	0	1	33	2.5	NA	Large toxicity, few	Wheeler [65]
BLEO+VCR+MMC +MTX	5	0	2	50	2.7,4	NA	pts, short responses	
BLEO+MTX	20	0	12	68	7.5	NA	Weekly BLEO	Conroy [66]
BLEO+MTX	8	3	2	63	3	4.3	No response or selection criteria	Piel [67]
BLEO+MTX+VCR +5FU+CTX+ ARA-C+ACT-D	18	0	8	44	4	NA	Toxic, no utility	Forney [68]

BLEO = Bleomycin; MMC = mitomycin-C; VCR = vincristine; MTX = methotrexate; 5FU = 5-fluorouracil; CTX = cyclophosphamide; Ara-C = cytosine arabinoside; ACT-D = actinomycin-D; CR = complete response; PR = partial response.

Based upon this large body of data, one may conclude that bleomycin-mitomycin-C probably has substantial activity in carcinoma of the cervix, depending upon the location of the tumor, the patient's ability to withstand the toxicity, and the aggressiveness of treatment. It is unfortunate that no randomized studies have been published to compare this combination with single agents. The short durations of response and survival of the two agents may not represent any improvement over those obtained with mitomycin, bleomycin, or adriamycin alone.

Other bleomycin combinations

Additional studies with bleomycin in combination with other agents are listed in Table 6. The studies of Baker *et al.* [61, 62] added vincristine to the Miyamoto regimen of bleomycin and mitomycin-C. The pilot study suggested activity [61] and was superceded by a large, randomized multiarm study of the Southwest Oncology Group (SWOG). The SWOG study tested the question of dosing and sequential therapy in the mitomycin-C-bleomycin regimen. The higher dose bleomycin-vincristine arm and the infusion bleomycin arm were thought to be equal, but the infusion arm was less toxic. All treatments resulted in substantial myelosuppression. Because of the short durations of response and survival, the authors recommended that the infusion regimen be considered for use early in the treatment of poor prognosis patients (neoadjuvant therapy). Treatment late in the course of the disease was considered too toxic for the benefits gained.

Other studies including vincristine, methotrexate, or mitomycin-C in various combinations do not show any promise for improvement in treatment results. The bleomycin-methotrexate combinations [66, 67], while claiming high response rates suffer from poor descriptions of patient selection criteria and little evidence of strict response criteria. It must be assumed that either extremely good prognosis patients were entered into these studies or response measurements were supoptimal, or both. The study of Forney *et al.* [68] is remarkable for the large number of drugs that patients were able to tolerate. It is likely that none of the drugs were administered in optimal doses, as that would have caused intolerable toxicity. Response rates and durations are no better than any previously reported data.

Cisplatin based combinations

Cisplatin added to bleomycin based combinations

The GOG [18] found a single agent response rate for cisplatin of approximately 25% in advanced cervix cancer. This represents an important order of activity. Investigators quickly added cisplatin to existing regimens to determine whether the addition of this drug could enhance response and survival rates (Tables 7 and 8).

ate.

Combination	Evaluable patients	CR	PR	Response (%)	Duration of response (median-months)	Survival (months)	Comments	Author (ref no.)
DDP+BLEO+MMC+VCR	13	3	7	78	4	10	Considered active, poor long-term survival, BLEO given weekly bolus	Vogl [69]
DDP+BLEO+MMC+VCR	14	4	2	43	14+	9	BLEO by infusion, long CR survival	Alberts [70]
DDP+BLEO+MMC+VCR	14	1	6	50	5.5	8	Very poor performances status	Giannone [71]
DDP+BLEO+MMC+VCR	14	1	2	21	4	4	Heterogeneous pt population, doses differed	Belinson [72]
DDP+BLEO+MMC+VCR	48	– 8 –		17	NA	NA	Heavy myelotoxicity. modest clinical benefit	Baker [73]
DDP+MMC	49	– 9 –		18				
DDP+BLEO	17	1	9	53	8	12.7	9 pts not prev treated	Block [74]
DDP+BLEO	24	0	13	54	3.5	6	No improvement in survival for responders	Daghestani [75]
DDP+BLEO+VBL	23	6	9	65	4.5–24	NA	Toxic, considered active 23-prev treatment,	Friedlander [76]
	10	0	6	60			10-no prev treatment	
DDP+MMC	30	3	10	43	12	12	22 pts had distant mets only	Pecorelli [77]
DDP+BLEO+MTX	19	0	10	53	4	9	Short resp duration and survival	Seltzer [78]
DDP+BLEO+VCR+MTX	15	3	7	66	7.3	12	Survival for responders only, myelotoxic	Rosenthal [79]
DDP+BLEO+VBL+MTX	5	0	0	–	–	–	Not useful	Leone [80]

DDP = cisplatin; BLEO = bleomycin; MMC = mitomycin-C; VCR = vincristine; MTX = methotrexate; VBL = vinblastine; CR = complete response; PR = partial response.

Table 8. Multiagent regimens including cisplatin in advanced cervix carcinoma: studies with new drugs, cyclophosphamide, and adriamycin.

Combination	Evaluable patients	CR	PR	Response (%)	Duration of response (median-months)	Survival (months)	Comments	Author (ref no.)
DDP+BLEO+ADR	21	4	4	38	9.5-CR	9.2	Distant mets responded	Sorbe [81]
DDP+CTX	12	2	3	42	6	NA	Optomistic pilot	Jobson [82]
DDP+DOX+MeCCNU	23	2	5	30	6	15+	Survivors for responders only, myelotoxic	Carlson [83]
DDP+DichloroMTX	13	6	4	76	12.3 CR 7 PR	18.8 CR 11.5 PR	Severe toxicity	Roberts [84]
DDP+CTX+ADR	20	1	3	20	9.5	NA	No better than DDP alone	Lele [85]
DDP+DAG	18	2	5	39	5	9	No better than DDP alone	Vogl [86]

DDP = cisplatin; BLEO = bleomycin; ADR = adriamycin; CTX = cyclophosphamide; MeCCNU = methyl-CCNU; DichloroMTX = dichloromethotrexate; DAG = dianhydrogalactitol; CR = complete response; PR = partial response.

Vogl *et al.* [69] initially reported data on their 'BOMP' combination. This combination was used with some success in head and neck patients. For cervix carcinoma, they reported a high response rate, substantial, but not intolerable toxicity, and poor response durations and survivals. In fact, these data do not appear much different from those obtained from mitomycin-C-bleomycin. Alberts *et al.* [70] gave bleomycin by a 4-day infusion instead of by a weekly injection at a dose of 10 mg/m^2/day for 4 days (MOB-P). While Alberts *et al.* reported a lower response rate, the durations of response and survivals were better. We have treated 14 patients with this regimen. Most of the patients in our series were bedridden. Fifty percent of our patients responded, but the responses were brief and survivals short [71].

The regimen of Alberts *et al.* [70] appears to be better tolerated than that of Vogl *et al.* The high complete response rate and longer survival time in the pilot study of Alberts *et al.* prompted a SWOG study (Baker *et al.* [72]) which has recently been reported in abstract form. The preliminary data are not promising and suggest a low order of activity for both MOB-P regimen and a control arm of cisplatin plus mitomycin-C. Both arms had substantial myelotoxicity and nephrotoxicity.

Additional studies of bleomycin and methotrexate combined with cisplatin are listed in Table 7. It appears that the combination of cisplatin-bleomycin [74, 75] has similar activity to other reported cisplatin containing regiments. Durations of response and survival are similar. The same may be said for the addition of methotrexate to cisplatin-bleomycin-mitomycin-C combinations. Cisplatin combinations including adriamycin, cyclophosphamide, and newer drugs (Table 8) produce similar data to those described above.

Summary and conclusions

Over the last 10 years, successive multiagent regimens based upon adriamycin, bleomycin, and cisplatin have been tested in patients with advanced carcinoma of the cervix. These agents alone induce responses in 15–30% of patients treated, although most treatment successes occur outside the pelvis. Since the pelvis is a major site of tumor recurrence and persistence, treatment with cytotoxic agents has not met with much success in improving survival of these patients.

Interpretation of different combination chemotherapy studies is made difficult by confusing response criteria, difficulties in measuring disease, different patient entry criteria, and different dose modification schedules for toxicity. Combination chemotherapy with the above agents plus most other commonly used cytotoxics has not greatly improved survival although response rates, including complete responses, have improved dramatically. It is unclear whether combination chemotherapy, with or without cisplatin is superior to single agent therapy using survival as the ultimate measurement of treatment success. Furthermore, in view of the recently presented Australian study of lung cancer treatment with and without chemotherapy [87], it can be questioned whether cytotoxic chemotherapy improves the survival outcome when compared to no treatment at all. It is evident that new agents and treatment approaches are necessary. Many of these new approaches are discussed in this volume.

Despite this pessimistic outlook, chemotherapy has demonstrated activity in this disease. This suggests that we do have some tools with which to treat advanced cervix cancer. A logical approach is to employ these tools when disease is at a minimal volume. Early chemotherapy prior to definitive debulking treatment with radiation or surgery (*neoadjuvant* treatment) has the theoretical advantage of delivering drug to the pelvis when the blood supply is not interrupted and the tumor has a minimum of resistant cells. Simultaneous drug treatment with radiation therapy may allow some of the cytotoxics to function as hypoxic cell sensitizers. These approachs may be useful in certain, as yet unidentified, subsets of patients and are worth investigating as we await newer, more innovative approaches to the treatment of solid tumors.

Acknowledgements

Supported by the Veterans Administration.

References

1. Clement PB, Scully RE. 1982. Carcinoma of the cervix: histologic types. Sem Oncol 9:251–264.
2. Tannock I. 1978. Cell kinetics and chemotherapy: A critical review. Cancer Treat Rep 62:1117–1133.
3. Glick JH, Marcial V, Richter M *et al.* 1980. The adjuvant treatment of inoperable stage II and IV epidermoid carcinoma of the head and neck with platinum and bleomycin infusions prior to definite radiotherapy. Cancer 46:1919–1924.
4. Spaulding M, Kahn A, De Los Santos R *et al.* 1982. Adjuvant chemotherapy in advanced head and neck cancer. Am J Surg 144:432–436.
5. Livingston RB. 1977. Combination chemotherapy of bronchogenic carcinoma. I. Non-oat cell. Cancer Treat Rev 4:153–165.
6. Nigro ND, Seydel HG, Considine B *et al.* 1983. Combined preoperative radiation and chemotherapy for squamous cell carcinoma of the anal canal. Cancer 51:1826–1829.
7. Kelsen DP, Coonley C, Bains M *et al.* 1983. Cisplatin, vindesine, and methyl-glyoxal bis (guanylhydrazone) combination chemotherapy of local-regional and advanced esophageal carcinoma. Am J Med 75:645–651.

8. Wasserman TH, Carter SK. 1977. The integration of chemotherapy into combined modality treatment of solid tumors. VIII. Cervical cancer. Cancer Treat Rev 4:25–46.
9. Morrow CP, DiSaia PJ, Mangan CF, Lagasse LD. 1977. Continuous pelvic arterial infusion with bleomycin for squamous carcinoma of the cervix recurrent after irradiation therapy. Cancer Treat Rep 61:1403–1405.
10. Swenerton KD, Evers JA, White GW, Boyes DA. 1979. Intermittent pelvic infusion with vincristine, bleomycin, and mitomycin C for advanced recurrent carcinoma of the cervix. Cancer Treat Rep 63:1379–1380.
11. Carlson JA, Freedman RS, Wallace S *et al.* 1974. Intraarterial cisplatinum in the management of squamous cell carcinoma of the cervix. Gynecol Oncol 12:92–98.
12. Kavanagh JJ, Rutledge F, Wharton J *et al.* 1982. Palliation of advanced recurrent pelvic malignancies by selective intraarterial combination chemotherapy. Proc Am Soc Clin Oncol 1:109.
13. Bonnadonna G, Valagussa P. 1981. Dose-response of adjuvant chemotherapy in breast cancer. N Engl J Med 304:10–15.
14. Van Nagell JR, Donaldson ES *et al.* 1978. Evaluation and treatment of patients with invasive cervical cancer. Surg Clin NA 58:67–85.
15. Brenner DE, Whitley NO, Villasanta U. 1982. An evaluation of the computed tomographic scanner for the staging of carcinoma of the cervix. Cancer 50:2327–2338.
16. Villasanta U, Whitley NO, Haney PJ, Brenner D. 1983. Computed tomography in invasive carcinoma of the cervix: An appraisal. Obstet Gynecol 63:218–224.
17. Brenner DE, Whitley NO, Houk T, Aisner J, Wiernik PH, Whitley J. 1982. Volume determinations by computed tomography. JAMA 247:1299–1302.
18. Thigpen T, Shingleton H, Homesley H, Lagasse L, Blessing J. 1981. Cis-platinum in treatment of advanced or recurrent squamous cell carcinoma of the cervix: A phase II study of the Gynecologic Oncology Group. Cancer 48:899–903.
19. Luria SE, Delbruck M. 1943. Mutations of bacteria from virus sensitivity to virus resistance. Genetics 28:491–511.
20. Goldie JH, Coldman AJ. 1979. A mathematic model for relating the drug sensitivity of tumors to the spontaneous mutation rate. Cancer Treat Rep 63:1727–1733.
21. Skipper HC, Chapman JB, Bell M. 1952. The anti-leukemic action of combinations of certain known anti-leukemia agents. Cancer Res 11:109–114.
22. DeVita VT. 1985. Principles of chemotherapy. In: Cancer, Principles and Practice of Oncology (VT DeVita, S Hellman, SA Rosenberg, eds). J.B. Lippincott, Philadelphia, pp 267–271.
23. Brenner DE. 1982. Carcinoma of the cervix: A review. Am J Med Sci 284:31–48.
24. Muscato MS, Perry MC, Yarbro JW. 1982. Chemotherapy of cervical carcinoma. Sem Oncol 9:373–387.
25. Thigpen T, Shingleton H, Homesley H, LaGasse L, Blessing J. 1979. Cis-dicholorodiamine-platinum (II) in the treatment of gynecologic malignancies. Phase II trials by the Gynecologic Oncology Group. Cancer Treat Rep 63:1549–1555.
26. Guthrie D, Way S. 1974. Treatment of advanced carcinoma of the cervix with adriamycin and methotrexate combined. Obstet Gynecol 44:586–589.
27. Guthrie D, Way S. 1978. The use of adriamycin and methotrexate in carcinoma of the cervix. Obstet Gynecol 52:349–354.
28. Haid M, Homesley HL, White DR *et al.* 1977. Adriamycin-methotrexate combination chemotherapy of advanced carcinoma of the cervix: A second look. Obstet Gynecol 50:103–105.
29. Papavasiliou G, Pappas J, Aravantinos D, Kaskarelis K. 1978. Treatment of cervical carcinoma with adriamycin combined with methotrexate. Cancer Treat Rep 62:1387–1388.
30. Piver MS, Barlow JJ, Xynos FP. 1978. Adriamycin alone or in combination in 100 patients with carcinoma of the cervix or vagina. Am J Obstet Gynecol 131:311–313.

31. Trope C, Johnsson JE, Grundsell H, Mattsson W. 1980. Adriamycin-methotrexate combination chemotherapy of advanced carcinoma of the cervix: a third look. Obstet Gynecol 55:488–492.
32. Maillot K, Ranger IM. 1982. Chemotherapy for advanced recurrent carcinoma of the cervix. Arch Gynecol 231:253–261.
33. Alberts DS, Ignoffo R. 1978. Adriamycin-cyclophosphamide treatment of squamous cell carcinoma of the cervix. Cancer Treat Rep 62:143–144.
34. Hanjani P, Bonnell S. 1980. Treatment of advanced and recurrent squamous cell carcinoma of the cervix with combination doxorubicin and cyclophosphamide. Cancer Treat Rep 64:1363–1365.
35. Wallace HJ, Hreshchyshyn MM, Wilbanks GD *et al.* 1978. Comparison of the therapeutic effects of adriamycin alone versus adriamycin plus vincristine versus adriamycin plus cyclophosphamide in the treatment of advanced carcinoma of the cervix. Cancer Treat Rep 62:1435–1441.
36. Sorbe B, Frankendal B. 1982. Combination chemotherapy in advanced carcinoma of the cervix. Cancer 50:2028–2030.
37. Piver MS, Barlow JJ, Dunbar J. 1980. Doxorubicin, cyclophosphamide, and 5-fluorouracil in patients with carcinoma of the cervix or vagina. Cancer Treat Rep 64:549–551.
38. Omura GA, Velez-Garcia E, Birch R. 1981. Phase II randomized study of doxorubicin, vincristine, and 5-FU versus cyclophosphamide in advanced squamous cell carcinoma of the cervix. Cancer Treat Rep 65:901–903.
39. Day TG, Wharton JT, Gottlieb JA, Rutledge FN. 1978. Chemotherapy for squamous carcinoma of the cervix: doxorubicin-methyl CCNU. Am J Obstet Gynecol 132:545–548.
40. Malkasian GD, Decker DG, Green SJ *et al.* 1981. Treatment of recurrent and metastatic carcinoma of the cervix: Comparison of doxorubicin with a combination of vincristine and 5-fluorouracil. Gynecol Oncol 11:235–239.
41. Hakes T, Nikrui M, Magill G, Ochoa M. 1979. Cervix cancer: Treatment with combination vincristine and high doses of methotrexate. Cancer 43:459–464.
42. Morrow CP, Creasman WT, DiSaia PJ *et al.* 1973. Methotrexate, hydroxyurea, and vincristine: Combination chemotherapy in squamous carcinoma of the female genetalia. Gynecol Oncol 1:314–319.
43. Akiyama S, Kuwano M. 1981. Isolation and preliminary characterization of bleomycin-resistant mutants from Chinese hamster ovary cells. J Cell Physiol 107:147–156.
44. de Palo GM, Bajetta E, Luciani L *et al.* 1973. Methotrexate and bleomycin in the treatment of advanced epidermoid carcinoma of the uterine cervix. Cancer Chemother Rep 57:429–435.
45. Barlow JJ, Piver MS, Chuang JT *et 1l.* 1973. Adriamycin and bleomycin alone and in combination in gynecologic cancers. Cancer 32:735–743.
46. Greenberg BR, Kardinal CG, Pajek TF, Bateman JR. 1977. Adriamycin versus adriamycin and bleomycin in advanced epidermoid carcinoma of the cervix. Cancer Treat Rep 61:1383–1384.
47. Terasima T, Takabe Y, Katsumata T *et al.* 1970. Effect of bleomycin on mammalian cell survival. J Natl Cancer Inst 49:1093–1100.
48. Tobey RA. 1975. Arrest of Chinese hamster cells in G2 following treatment with the antitumor drug bleomycin. J Cell Physiol 79:259–266.
49. Miyamoto T, Takabe Y, Watanabe M, Terasima T. 1978. Effectiveness of a sequential combination of bleomycin and mitomycin-C on advanced cervical cancer. Cancer 41:403–414.
50. Barranco SC, Luce SK, Ramsdahl MW *et al.* 1973. Bleomycin as a possible synchronizing agent for human tumor cells in vivo. Cancer Res 33:882–887.
51. Shimoyama M, Kimura K. 1972. Quantitative clonal growth of mammalian cells: Its application for quantitative study of cytocidal action of mitomycin-C. Gann 63:773–783.

52. Miyamoto T. 1980. Recent results of using a sequential combination of bleomycin and mitomycin-C in the treatment of metastatic cervical cancer. In: Recent Results in Cancer Research Research (70) New Anticancer Drugs (SK Carter, Y Sakurai, eds). Springer-Verlag, New York, pp 211–217.
53. Llorens AS. 1980. Chemotherapy of squamous cell carcinoma of the cervix. Obstet Gynecol 55:373–375.
54. Krebbs HB, Girtanner RE, Nordqvist SRB *et al.* 1980. Treatment of advanced cervical cancer by combination of bleomycin and mitomycin-C. Cancer 46:2159–2161.
55. Leichman LP, Baker LH, Stanhope CR *et al.* Mitomycin-C and bleomycin in the treatment of far-advanced cervical cancer: A Southwest Oncology Group pilot study. Cancer Treat Rep 64:1139–1140.
56. Boice CR, Freedman RS, Herson J *et al.* 1982. Bleomycin and Mitomycin-C in recurrent squamous uterine cervical carcinoma. Cancer 49:2242–2245.
57. Petrilli ES, Castaldo TW, Ballon SC *et al.* 1980. Bleomycin-mitomycin C therapy for advanced squamous carcinoma of the cervix. Gynecol Oncol 9:292–297.
58. Greenberg BR, Hannigan J, Gerretson L *et al.* 1982. Sequential combination of bleomycin and mitomycin-C in advanced cervical cancer. An American experience: A Northern California Oncology Group Study. Cancer Treat Rep 66:163–165.
59. Trope C, Johnsson JE, Simonsen E *et al.* 1983. Bleomycin-mitomycin C in advanced carcinoma of the cervix: A third look. Cancer 51:591–593.
60. Copas P, Dyer M, Smithson LG, Hall DJ. 1983. Bleomycin-mitomycin C in advanced squamous cell carcinoma of the female genital tract. Obstet Gynecol 61:308–310.
61. Baker LH, Opipari MI, Izbicki RM. 1976. Phase II study of mitomycin-C, vincristine, and bleomycin in advanced squamous cell carcinoma of the uterine cervix. Cancer 38:2222–2224.
62. Baker LH, Opipari MI, Wilson H, Bottomley R, Coltman CA. 1977. Mitomycin C, vincristine, and bleomycin therapy for advanced cervical cancer. Obstet Gynecol 52:146–150.
63. Behnam K, Lewis GC, Lee JH, Looka MH. 1981. Treatment of cervical carcinoma with methotrexate, bleomycin and vincristine. Cancer Clin Trials 4:74–79.
64. Hannigan EV, Dillard EA, Dinh TV. 1984. Bleomycin, vincristine, and methotrexate with citrovorum factor rescue in the treatment of advanced squamous cell carcinoma of the cervix. Gynecol Oncol 19:57–59.
65. Wheeler RH, Liepman MK, Baker SR *et al.* 1980. Bleomycin, vincristine, and mitomycin-C with or without methotrexate in the treatment of squamous cell carcinoma. Cancer Treat Rep 64:943–949.
66. Conroy JF, Lewis GC, Brady LW *et al.* 1976. Low dose bleomycin and methotrexate in cervical cancer. Cancer 37:660–664.
67. Piel IJ, Slayton RE, Perlia CP, Wilbanks GD. 1973. Combination chemotherapy with bleomycin and methotrexate in recurrent and disseminated cervical carcinoma: A preliminary study. Gynecol Oncol 1:184–190.
68. Forney JP, Morrow CP, DiSaia PJ, Futoran RJ. 1975. Seven-drug polychemotherapy in the treatment of advanced and recurrent squamous carcinoma of the female genital tract. Am J Obstet Gynecol 123:748–752.
69. Vogl SE, Moukhtar M, Calanog A *et al.* 1980. Chemotherapy for advanced cervical cancer with bleomycin, vincristine, mitomycin C, and cis-diamminedichloroplatinum (II) (BOMP). Cancer Treat Rep 64:1005–1007.
70. Alberts DS, Martimbeau PW, Surwit EA, Oishi N. 1981. Mitomycin-C, bleomycin, Vincristine, and cis-Platinum in the treatment of advanced recurrent squamous cell carinoma of the cervix. Cancer Clin Trials 4:313–316.
71. Giannone L, Brenner DE, Jones HW, Greco FA, Burnett LS. Combination chemotherapy for patients with advanced carcinoma of the cervix: Trial of mitomycin-C, vincristine, bleomycin, and cisplatin. Gynecol Oncol (in press).

72. Belinson JL, Stewart JA, Richards AL, McClure M. 1985. Bleomycin, vincristine, mitomysin-C, and cisplatin in the management of gynecological squamous cell carcinomas. Gynecol Oncol 20:387–393.
73. Baker L, Boutselis J, Alberts D, Surwit E, Hilgers R. 1985. Combination chemotherapy for patients with disseminated carcinoma of the uterine cervix. Proc Am Soc Clin Oncol 4:120.
74. Bloch B, Nel CP, Kriel A *et al.* 1984. Combination chemotherapy with cisplatin and bleomycin in advanced cervical cancer. Cancer Treat Rep 68:891–893.
75. Daghestani AN, Hakes TB, Lynch G, Lewis JL. 1983. Cervix carcinoma: Treatment with combination cisplatin and bleomycin. Gynecol Oncol 16:334–339.
76. Friedlander M, Kaye SB, Sullivan A *et al.* 1983. Cervical carcinoma: A drug responsive tumor-experience with combined cisplatin, vinblastine, and bleomycin therapy. Gynecol Oncol 16:275–281.
77. Pecorelli S, Mangioni C, van der Burg MEL *et al.* 1985. Phase II study of mitomycin C and cisplatin in disseminated squamous cell carcinoma of the uterine cervix. Proc Am Soc Clin Oncol 4:115.
78. Seltzer V, Vogl SE, Davis TE, Camacho F. 1985. Chemotherapy of cervical cancer with cisplatinum, bleomycin, and standard dose methotrexate with leucovorin rescue-a safe program with limited activity. Proc Am Soc Clin Oncol 4:123.
79. Rosenthal CJ, Khulpateea N, Boyce J *et al.* 1983. Effective chemotherapy for advanced carcinoma of the cervix with bleomycin, cisplatin, vincristine, and methotrexate. Cancer 52:2025–2030.
80. Leone L, Rege V, Schilling A, Miller B. 1985. Treatment of advanced squamous gynecologic neoplasms. Proc Am Soc Clin Oncol 4:120.
81. Sorbe B, Frankeldal B. 1984. Bleomycin-adriamycin-cisplatin combination chemotherapy in the treatment of primary advanced and recurrent cervical carcinoma. Obstet Gynecol 63:167–171.
82. Jobson VW, Muss HB, Thigpen JT *et al.* 1984. Chemotherapy of advanced squamous carcinoma of the cervix: A phase I-II study of high-dose cisplatin and cyclophosphamide. Am J Clin Oncol 7:341–345.
83. Carlson JA, Day TG, Allegra JC *et al.* 1984. Methyl-CCNU, doxorubicin, and cisdiamine-dicholoplatinum II in the management of recurrent and metastatic squamous carcinoma of the cervix. Cancer 54:211–214.
84. Roberts JA, Morley GW, Natale RB, Wheeler RH. 1984. Combination cisplatin and dichloromethotrexate in patients with advanced or recurrent cervical cancer: A preliminary report. Gynecol Oncol 19:194–197.
85. Lele SB, Piver MS, Barlow JJ. 1983. Cyclophosphamide, adriamycin, and platinum chemotherapy in treatment of advanced and recurrent cervical carcinoma. Gynecol Oncol 16: -15–18.
86. Vogl SE, Seltzer V, Camacho F, Calanog A. 1982. Dianhydrogalactitol and cisplatin in combination for advanced cancer of the uterine cervix. Cancer Treat Rep 66:1809–1812.
87. Woods RL, Levi JA, Page J *et al.* 1985. Non small cell cancer: A randomized comparison of chemotherapy with no chemotherapy. Proc Am Soc Clin Oncol 4:177.

11. Primary chemotherapy for high-risk recurrence cervix cancer

DAVID S. ALBERTS, SILVIO ARISTIZABAL,
EARL A. SURWIT and SHELDON WEINER

Introduction

As has been discussed in previous chapters patients with lymph node positive, stages I and II and advanced stages III and IV cervix cancer have poor prognoses, regardless of local treatment type (Tables 1 and 2, respectively). For example, the 5-year survival rate has been reported to be as low as 54% in patients with lymph node positive, stage IB disease [1] and 30–40% in patients with bulky, stage III disease [2]. Recurrences in these high-risk groups occur both locally and distally in similar frequencies. The utilization of more aggressive regional therapy techniques in advanced disease as described by Aristizabal *et al.* in an earlier chapter has been associated with significantly higher control rates of local disease, but patients continue to die from systemic metastases. Clearly, new multimodality treatment programs must be directed toward the sterilization of both bulky, localized disease and distant, microscopic metastases.

One relatively recent innovation in cancer management has been the use of chemotherapy as initial treatment prior to surgery or radiation therapy in patients with advanced stage head and neck tumors and osteogenic sarcomas. As will be described, the results of treatment demonstrate that pro-

Table 1. The influence of primary tumor category on survival (effect of lymph node involvement).

	Percentage 5-year survival rate	
Stage	Node negative	Node positive
I B	91	54
II A	67	28

Modified from Piver and Chung, 1975 [1].

E.A. Surwit, D.S. Alberts (eds) Cervix Cancer.
 ISBN 0-89838-822-8. Printed in the Netherlands.

Table 2. Results of treatment of cervix cancer by definitive radiation therapy.

<table>
<tr><th rowspan="2">Investigators</th><th rowspan="2">Total cases</th><th colspan="2">Stage I</th><th colspan="2">Stage II</th><th colspan="2">Stage III</th><th rowspan="2">Stage IV</th></tr>
<tr><th>A</th><th>B</th><th>A</th><th>B</th><th>A</th><th>B</th></tr>
<tr><td>Brand and Kerr, 1982 [a]</td><td>1059</td><td></td><td>75</td><td>75</td><td></td><td colspan="2">40</td><td>8</td></tr>
<tr><td>Jampolis et al., 1975</td><td>924</td><td></td><td>91</td><td>82</td><td>65</td><td>54</td><td>40</td><td>–</td></tr>
<tr><td>Jiminez et al., 1979</td><td>1227</td><td colspan="2">81</td><td>56</td><td></td><td colspan="2">36</td><td>12</td></tr>
<tr><td>Perez et al., 1983 [b]</td><td>849</td><td></td><td>87</td><td>73</td><td>68</td><td colspan="2">44</td><td>0</td></tr>
</table>

[a] Actuarial survival.
[b] NED.
Modified from Langlands and Hudson, 1985 [2].

longed disease-free survival depends directly on the degree of reduction of the bulky primary tumor by induction chemotherapy. The rationale for primary chemotherapy (i.e. anticancer drug treatment prior to definitive surgery and/or radiation therapy) in patients with advanced and/or high-risk of recurrence cancers includes the following:

1. improved drug distribution into untreated tumors with an intact vascularity, rather than to tumors that have been exposed to surgery or radiation;
2. better tolerance of intensive chemotherapy in previously untreated patients with good performance and nutritional statuses;
3. enhanced efficacy of the planned definitive local treatment after cytoreduction of the primary tumor and nodal mestastases;
4. possible eradication of subclinical metastases [3].

For these reasons, several groups of investigators have initiated trials of primary chemotherapy in patients with previously untreated, advanced cervix cancer. In this chapter we will review the results of primary chemotherapy in patients with head and neck cancer and osteogenic sarcoma prior to describing the more preliminary data from similar trials in patients with high-risk of recurrence squamous cell cancers of the cervix.

Primary chemotherapy of head and neck cancer

Advanced stage III and IV squamous cell cancers of the head and neck are incurable in the vast majority of patients treated with standard surgery and radiation therapy, either alone or in combination [4, 5]. Because of the poor prognosis of patients with advanced disease primary chemotherapy trials were begun in the mid to late 1970s. Initially these trials utilized combinations of cisplatin and bleomycin and were associated with clinical complete response rates of 20 to 30% prior to surgery or radiation therapy [6, 7].

More recently, investigators at Wayne State University have carried out two consecutive trials with a combination of cisplatin and 5-fluorouracil (5FU). In the first of these studies, 5FU was administered in a dose of 1 gm/m^2 daily for four consecutive days by continuous infusion after cisplatin, 100 mg/m^2 on day 1. Although the overall objective response rate was 88% after two courses of chemotherapy the clinical complete response rate was only 19% [8]. It is of extreme interest that the extension of the 5FU infusion to 5 days (from 4) and the addition of a third course of chemotherapy resulted in a 56% complete response rate prior to surgery and/or radiation therapy [8]. This significant increase in complete response ($p = 0.04$) indicates that more intensive and prolonged primary chemotherapy is likely to lead to higher rates of complete tumor disappearance.

Forty-one percent of the complete remitters in the Wayne State trials [9], were alive at 36 months of follow-up as compared to only 5% survivors in the group of patients who experienced only partial responses to chemotherapy. Unfortunately, differences in the type of chemotherapy, amount of radiation and patient sex did not explain the prolonged survival in the complete responders.

Conclusions concerning primary chemotherapy in the management of previously untreated, advanced head and neck cancers include the following:

1. patients who experience a complete response to chemotherapy survive significantly longer than partial or non-responders;
2. the percentage of patients enjoying improved survival increases when the percentage of complete response to chemotherapy increases;
3. thus far, there is no convincing evidence that primary chemotherapy can improve the survival of the entire treated patient group;
4. it is obvious that only well controlled, randomized trials will prove that primary chemotherapy can significantly impact on the overall survival durations of these patients.

Primary chemotherapy of osteogenic sarcoma

Investigators at Memorial Sloan-Kettering Cancer Center in New York City have reported their more than 10-year experience using primary chemotherapy in the management of patients with previously untreated osteogenic sarcoma [10]. During this period, Rosen and his group have treated 206 patients with pre-operative chemotherapy with the purpose of chemically debulking localized disease and eradicating potential, distant micrometastases.

The chemotherapy in the first 155 patients consisted of pre-operative high dose methotrexate with leucovorin rescue plus cyclophosphamide or the combination of bleomycin, cyclophosphamide, dactinomycin (BCD) plus doxorubicin or doxorubicin in combination with cisplatin [11]. A later trial consisted of high dose methotrexate plus BCD without doxorubicin. Patients that had a good response to preoperative chemotherapy had termination of chemotherapy one month after definitive surgery. In general, a good response to preoperative chemotherapy was defined as > 90% of the resected primary tumor showing no evidence of viable tumor on histologic examination. Only occasional microscopic foci of viable appearing tumor cells were allowed in this category of response. A poor response to preoperative chemotherapy was defined as any one section from the resected primary tumor showing confluent areas of viable appearing tumor cells.

Of the entire 206 patients in this series, 48% had a good response to chemotherapy based on histologic evaluation and 52% had a poor response. Of the 98 patients who had a good response, 91% have experienced continuous disease-free survival, and 96% were alive as of 1984. Nine treatment failures following a good response to chemotherapy included four patients with local recurrences, three patients with a solitary lung metastases, one patient with a soft tissue metastases, and one patient who died of varicella while undergoing treatment.

The overall end results of pre-operative chemotherapy for osteogenic sarcoma over the last decade at Memorial Sloan-Kettering Cancer Center reveals a cure rate of 81% and a relapse free survival rate of 75%. Several conclusions can be drawn from these pre-operative chemotherapy trials, including the following:

1. the more intensive the chemotherapy regimen, the greater the likelihood of both good response and prolonged disease-free survival. For example, the escalation of the methotrexate dose from 8 g/m^2 to 12 g/m^2 in fully grown adolescents and adults resulted in significantly improved good response rates and prolonged disease-free survival;
2. a good response of the primary tumor to chemotherapy is associated with a high likelihood of long-term disease-free survival. Conversely, patients whose primary tumor failed to respond favorably to chemotherapy also failed to remain continuously free of disease, regardless of the type or duration of postoperative adjuvant chemotherapy;
3. in the setting of primary chemotherapy of osteogenic sarcoma it appears that eradication of the primary tumor is also associated with the sterilization of potential micrometastases. Of course, this is an important conclusion for primary chemotherapy of various types of solid tumors;
4. it appears that even a complete histologic response to chemotherapy of the primary osteogenic sarcoma is not sufficient to prevent a local recurrence if radical surgery is not performed. Thus, an overall conclusion for primary chemotherapy of solid tumors is that definitive surgery or radiation therapy must be completed if sterilization of the primary tumor is to be achieved.

Chemotherapy for advanced cervix cancer

Single agent therapy

In a previous chapter Dr Tate Thigpen discussed the activity of single anticancer agents in the treatment of advanced, recurrent squamous cell cancer of the cervix. As concluded by Dr Thigpen, cisplatin appears to be the single most active agent in the management of these patients. Unfortunately, complete responses are uncommon and the median duration of response is less than 6 months. In the near future it is unlikely that any new cytotoxic agent or biologic modifier used alone will prove significantly more active than cisplatin in the treatment of this relatively drug resistant disease.

Recently, Bonomi *et al.* [12] reported the results of a randomized trial of three different cisplatin dosing schedules in the treatment of recurrent and/or metastatic cervix cancer. Although no one of the three cisplatin dosing regimens (i.e. 50 mg/m^2 on day 1 vs. 100 mg/m^2 on day 1 vs. 20 mg/m^2 for 5 consecutive days) was associated with a significantly better complete remission rate or response or survival duration, the 100 mg/m^2 dose administered every 21 days did induce a significantly better overall response rate ($p = 0.015$). These data taken together with the well-documented dose-response relationship associated with cisplatin *in vitro* against human tumor clonogenic cells [13] suggest that the 100 mg/m^2 dosing regimen should be selected for future primary chemotherapy trials in patients with advanced cervix cancer.

Combination chemotherapy

In the previous chapter, Dr Dean Brenner outlined in detail the efficacy of various combinations of cytotoxic agents which have been used to treat the recurrent and/or metastatic squamous cell cancers of the cervix. Virtually all of these combinations have been associated with relatively low clinical complete response rates and none of them have prolonged survival duration of the entire treated group. Most responses to single agent or combination chemotherapy regimens are observed in patients with metastases to lymph nodes, soft tissue or lung parenchyma. Chemotherapy of any type has been associated rarely with significant reductions in the size of previously irradiated pelvic tumor masses. Indeed, an immediate sign that a new chemotherapeutic approach may be promising is the observation of a relatively high response rate of pelvic disease.

Clearly, the major impetus to evaluate primary chemotherapy programs in patients with advanced cancer to the cervix relates to the initial success of primary chemotherapy of bulky, stage III and IV squamous cell cancers of the head and neck. The high complete response rates observed with primary chemotherapy of patients with advanced head and neck cancers suggests that similar therapeutic approaches in advanced cancer of the cervix might successfully reduce the size of bulky pelvic tumors as well as sterilize distant micrometastatic disease. Because of documented cross-resistance between radiation therapy and many anticancer agents and the adverse effect of radiation therapy on the distribution of drugs into pelvic tumors, it is unlikely that any chemotherapeutic approach will prove useful in patients with recurrent disease following primary surgery and/or radiation therapy. Thus, a good rationale exists for the development of primary chemotherapy trials to evaluate both new cytotoxic agents, biologic modifiers and various drug combinations in the setting of patients with previously untreated, advanced pelvic tumors. The remainder of this chapter will deal with the initial trials of primary chemotherapy in the setting of patients with advanced, previously untreated cervix cancer.

Primary chemotherapy in previously untreated, advanced cervix cancer

Systemic chemotherapy trials (Table 3)

Friedlander *et al.* [14] treated 30 patients (FIGO stages IB –6%, IIA – 17%, IIB – 30%, IIIA – 17%, and IIIB – 30%) with chemotherapy followed by either surgery or radiotherapy. The chemotherapeutic regimen consisted of: cisplatin (60 mg/m^2 IV, day 1), vinblastine (4 mg/m^2 IV, days 1 and 2), and bleomycin (15 mg IM, days 1, 8, and 15) administered every 3 weeks for a maximum of three courses. Seventeen percent of the patients had a complete clinical response to chemotherapy (i.e., disappearance of all disease) and 50% had a partial response to chemotherapy (i.e., decrease equal to or greater than 50% of the product of the maximal tumor diameters), yielding an overall response rate of 67%. Twenty-three percent had stable disease after chemotherapy. In nine patients (5 CR, 4 PR) radical hysterectomy and lymphadenectomy were performed following chemotherapy. All five patients with a clinical complete response were found to have microscopic disease at surgery. The four patients with a partial response had macroscopic disease present at surgery. These nine patients were reported alive with no evidence of disease for a median follow-up of 28+ weeks (range 20+ – 52+ weeks). Twenty-one patients were treated with radiation therapy immediately following chemotherapy. Of the 18 patients who completed radiation therapy and were evaluable for survival duration, ten had experienced a partial response and seven had stable disease following chemotherapy. Six of the ten patients with a partial response were alive with no evidence of recurrence for a median follow-up duration of 70+ weeks (range 26+ –

Table 3. Published studies of primary chemotherapy of advanced cervix cancer – systemic chemotherapy trials.

Reference	No. of patients	Disease stages	Chemotherapy regimen	No. of courses	Response to chemotherapy	Response duration	Survival duration
Friedlander *et al.*, Australia, 1983, followed by radiation therapy or surgery	30	IB 6% IIA 17% IIB 30% IIIA 17% IIIB 30%	Bleo 15 mg IM D1, 8, 15 VLB 4 mg/m^2 IV D1–2 every 3 wks PLAT 60 mg/m^2 IV D1 every 3 wks	3 cycles maximum	CR (5) 17% PR (15) 50% SD (7) 23% PD (3) 10%	After surgery: 9 patients NED 20+-52+ wks After radiation: 18 patients 9 NED 26+-156+ wks 3 dead NED 3 dead with disease	Not stated
Hakes *et al.*, MS-KCC 1984, followed by radiation therapy	30	IB 90% IIA 10% (high risk for recurrence)	Bleo 20 u/m^2 IV bolus D1, every 3–4 wks 20 u/m^2 × 3d continuous infusion D2–4 Cis PLAT 75 mg/m^2 D4 every 3–4 wks	2 2 2	Not stated	After radiation: Median = 20+ mos mean follow up 20.5 mos+ 5 recurrences	Not stated
Valle *et al.*, Brazil, 1985, followed by surgery – more chemotherapy	17	IIIA & B	Adria 50 mg/m^2 IV every 3wks Bleo 10 mg/d × 5d IV every 3 wks PLAT 100 mg/m^2 IV every 3 wks	Before surgery (3–5) After surgery (6–8)	CR (5) 29% PR (10) 59%	After surgery: 12 patients CR 11.5+ mos 50% NED; 25 mos	17+ mos
	18	IIIA & B	Adria 50 mg/m^2 IV every 3 wks Bleo 6 mg/d × 5d PLAT 50 mg/d × 5d	Before surgery (3–5) After surgery (6–8)	CR (3) 17% PR (10) 55%	After surgery: 12 patients CR 7.4+ mos 92% NED; 15 mos	15+ mos

Table 3. (Continued).

Reference	No. of patients	Disease stages	Chemotherapy regimen	No. of courses	Response to chemotherapy	Response duration	Survival duration
Smith *et al.*, Seattle, 1985, followed by radiation therapy	8	IB 12.5% IIA 12.5% IIB 37.5% IIIB 37.5%	Allopurinol 300 mg po every 8 h, D1–6 MTX 200 mg/m^2 IV D2 5FU 800 mg/m^2 IV (24 h infusion) D2–5 Leucovorin 20 mg IV 24 h after MTX, 20 mg after IV every 6 h × 16 PLAT 100 mg/m^2 IV, D4	(1–6)	CR 50% PR 50%	After radiation: 6 patients 5 NED; 1 LWD	Too early
Fine *et al.*, Princess Margaret Hospital, Toronto, 1983	5	Adv. Ca	MTX 40 mg/m^2 IV every 3wks Doxorubicin 50 mg/m^2 IV every 3 wks PLAT 50 mg/m^2 IV every 3 wks	Not stated	100% CR+PR	4+–24+ mos	4+–24+ mos
Belinson *et al.*, Vermont, 1984	2	IIIB, IV	Bleo 15 u/^{2}/d IV, D1–3 every 4wks VCR 1.4 mg/m^2 IV D3 every 4 wks MIT C 10 mg/m^2 IV D3 every other cycle PLAT 60 mg/m^2 IV D3 every 4 wks	3–4	CR (1) 50% PR (1) 50%	3 mos 1 mo	1 alive (15+ mos) 1 dead (6 mos)

Table 3. (Continued).

Reference	No. of patients	Disease stages	Chemotherapy regimen	No. of courses	Response to chemotherapy	Response duration	Survival duration
Kavanagh *et al.**, M.D. Anderson Hospital & Tumor Institute, Houston, 1983	10	III B IV A	Bleo 25–30 mg/m^2 IA continuous infusion every 3 wks Mit-C 10 mg/m^2 IA 4 h infusion every 3 wks PLAT 100 mg/m^2 IA 24 h continuous infusion every 3wks VCR 2 mg IV every 3 wks	3	60% response, 4 had biopsy conversion from malignant to non malignant status	Not stated	Not stated
Scarabelli *et al.**, Italy, 1985, followed by surgery or radiation	10	II B 20% III B 60% IV A 10% ? 10%	Peptichemio 20 mg IA every 5 days Doxorubicin 10 mg IA every 5 days PLAT 20 mg IA every 5 days	5–6 5–6	CR 20% PR 70%	Not stated	Range 9+–25+ mos

104+ weeks). Three others who were clinically disease-free died shortly after completing radiotherapy. Three of the seven patients with stable disease had no evidence of disease for a median follow-up of 52+ weeks (range 32+ - 156+ weeks). The other four patients relapsed within a year of completing radiotherapy.

Hakes *et al.* [15] studied 30 patients with stages IB (90%) and IIA (10%) disease who were at high risk for recurrence. These patients were given a regimen beginning 7–14 days after surgical diagnosis and staging consisting of: bleomycin (20 units/m^2 IV bolus on day 1 followed by 20 units/m^2 by continuous infusion on days 2–4) and cisplatin (75 mg/m^2 on day 4) given every 3–4 weeks for 2–3 courses of treatment. Chemotherapy was followed by external radiation therapy (4000–4200 rads to the pelvis). Median follow-up duration was 20+ months (range 3+ - 36+ months) with five recurrences (four local, one distant followed by local). The recurrences were observed at a median follow-up duration of 8 months (range 7–13 months). Survival durations and long-term follow-up of recurrent disease patients were not reported.

Valle *et al.* [16] reported their findings in 35 cervix cancer patients (stages IIIA and IIIB) given primary chemotherapy followed by surgery and further adjuvant chemotherapy. In seventeen patients chemotherapy consisted of: doxorubicin (50 mg/m^2), bleomycin (10 mg/day $\times$ 5 days) and cisplatin (100 mg/m^2) repeated every 3 weeks for 3–5 cycles of treatment. Due to unacceptable toxicity, the remaining 18 patients were treated with: doxorubicin (50 mg/m^2), bleomycin (6 mg/day $\times$ 5 days), and cisplatin (50 mg/m^2) repeated every 3 weeks for 3–5 cycles. The overall response rate prior to surgery was 88% (CR in five patients or 29%, PR in ten patients or 59%) in the group of 17 patients who received the higher dose of chemotherapy. In the low dose group of 18 patients the overall response rate was 72% (CR in three patients or 17%, PR in ten patients or 55%). A modified radical hysterectomy was performed on 12 of the 15 responders in the high dose group and of those 12, two patients had pathologically proven complete response. The remaining ten had residual disease. In the low dose group, 12 of the 13 responders underwent surgery. A complete response was proven in three patients and residual disease was found in the other nine. The patients' adjuvant chemotherapy consisted of the same regimen administered prior to surgery for a total of 6–8 cycles. The 12 patients in the high dose group had a median disease-free survival duration of 11.5+ months and a median survival duration of 17+ months. At 25 months, six patients (50%) had no evidence of disease, two had relapsed and four had died. The 12 patients in the low dose group had a median disease-free survival duration of 7.4+ months. At 15 months, all 12 of these patients were alive. Eleven patients (92%) were disease-free and one patient had recurrent disease.

Smith *et al.* [17] treated eight patients with advanced cervical cancer (FIGO stage IB or higher) with chemotherapy consisting of: allopurinol (300 mg every 8 h PO daily for 6 days), methotrexate (200 mg/m^2 IV, day 2), 5-FU (800 mg/m^2 24 h continuous infusion starting 1 h after methotrexate, days 2, 3, 4, and 5) leucovorin (20 mg IV 24 h after methotrextate followed by 20 mg every 6 h ×16 doses PO or IV, days 3, 4, 5 and 6), and cisplatin (100 mg/m^2 IV, day 4) given every 3 weeks for a median of 3 courses (range 1–6 courses) prior to radiation. Following radiation, chemotherapy was continued for two more courses if periaortic nodes had biopsy proven microscopic disease. The overall response rate prior to radiation for all patients was 100% (CR in four patients or 50%, PR in four patients or 50%). Of six patients who had completed radiotherapy, five had no evidence of disease with a median follow-up duration of 3+ months (range 2+ – 6+ months). Long-term response and survival duration data have not been reported.

Fine *et al.* [18] reported their findings in five patients with advanced cervix cancers treated with: methotrexate (40 mg/m^2 IV), doxorubicin (50 mg/m^2 IV), and cisplatin (50 mg/m^2 IV) given every 3 weeks for an unreported number of courses. All five patients (100%) responded to chemotherapy and were reported alive without clinical evidence of recurrence for 4+ to 24+ months.

Belinson *et al.* [19] studied two patients with a chemotherapeutic regimen consisting of: bleomycin (15 units/m^2/day IV, days 1, 2, and 3 by continuous infusion), vincristine (1.4 mg/m^2 IV, day 3), mitomycin-C (10 mg/m^2 IV, day 3), and cisplatin (60 mg/m^2 IV, day 3) repeated every 4 weeks with the exception of mitomycin-C which was repeated every other cycle. The median number of courses given was 3.5. One patient had radiation therapy following chemotherapy. One of the two patients who had stage IIIB disease had a complete response lasting 3 months and has survived 15+ months following radiation therapy. The second patient who had stage IV disease had a short duration (1 month) partial response to chemotherapy and survived only 6 months.

Intra-arterial chemotherapy trials (Table 3)

Kavanaugh *et al.* [20] treated ten patients (FIGO stages IIIB and IVA) with intra-arterial (IA) chemotherapy consisting of: vincristine (2 mg IV), mitomycin-C (10 mg/m^2 IA over 4 h), bleomycin (25–80 mg/m^2 IA over 24 h), and cisplatin (100 mg/m^2 IA over 24 h) given every 3 weeks for three courses. Of the ten patients treated with this regimen, there were six (60%) responders (i.e., 50% or 'substantial' reduction in tumor bulk, pain relief, cessation of vaginal bleeding, and significant improvement on angiography and computerized tomography). Four of the six responders had biopsy proven conversion from malignant to non-malignant status. However, local recurrence rates and survival data were not reported.

Scarabelli *et al.* [21] reported their results in ten patients with advanced cervix cancer (FIGO stages IIB, IIIB, and IVA) treated with intra-arterial therapy consisting of: peptichemio (20 mg IA), doxorubicin (10 mg IA), and cisplatin (20 mg IA) given over 5 h every 5 days for 5–6 cycles. Patients were subsequently treated with surgery or radiation therapy. The overall response rate to chemotherapy prior to subsequent treatment was 90% (CR in two patients or 20%, PR in seven patients or 70%). The complete responses were pathologically proven at the time of surgery. No response durations were stated, but survival durations ranged from 9+ – 25+ months.

Arizona Cancer Center trials (Tables 4–10)

The Arizona Cancer Center and the Southwest Oncology Group completed a pilot study to evaluate the activity of the MOB plus cisplatin regimen (see 'Treatment administration and dosing schedule for MOB plus cisplatin' on following pages) in patients with squamous cell cancers of the cervix, recurrent after pelvic irradiation or with distant metastases [22]. Of 14 evaluable patients there were three complete responders (21%) and four partial responders (29%). Two of the complete responders had complete disappearance of lung metastases and have remained free-of-disease for 7+ years. The third complete responder had experienced progression of her stage IIIB disease during intensive pelvic irradiation. The large pelvic mass regressed completely following two courses of MOB plus cisplatin therapy and she remained disease-free for four years. Despite a pelvic recurrence she remains alive at 7+ years after initial chemotherapy. Because of the apparent activity of the MOB plus cisplatin regimen against both local and distant disease and the unusually prolonged complete response durations, we initiated a trial of primary chemotherapy with two courses of the MOB plus cisplatin followed by definitive radiation therapy in patients with previously untreated, advanced cervix cancers [23].

Patients

Patients were eligible for this study if they had previously untreated epidermoid carcinoma of the cervix, either stage I or II disease with biopsy confirmed node metastases or stage III or IV disease. Patients with visceral metastases were excluded. Patients could not have received cytotoxic chemotherapy or treatment with radiation to the pelvis or abdomen. Patients were 65 years of age or younger with a life expectancy of at least 6 months.

All patients had a Southwest Oncology Group performance status (PS) of 0–2 (i.e., Karnofsky PS of 70–100) and adequate renal function at the time of drug initiation (i.e. BUN < 25 mg %, creatinine < 1.6 mg %). Patients with uncontrolled active sites of infection (i.e., fistula, abcess, etc.) or prior malignancies were also excluded. To be eligible for study, all patients signed an institutionally reviewed consent form written according to Federal guidelines.

All patients had baseline history and physical examinations, accurate clinical staging of cervical cancer, complete blood cell (CBC) counts, platelet count, renal panel and liver function tests. An initial IVP or CAT scan of the abdomen and pelvis and chest roentgenogram were obtained. During chemotherapy or radiation, CBCs and platelet counts were obtained weekly and PS was evaluated every 3 weeks. Prior to each course of chemotherapy, all pretreatment chemistries were repeated. After the completion of chemotherapy or radiation, the chest roentgenogram and IVP were repeated every six months. All other radiographs were obtained as indicated.

Treatment administration and dosing schedule for MOB plus cisplatin

The starting doses for all patients were:

- vincristine: 0.5 mg/m^2 IV on days 1 and 4 for two cycles only every 6 weeks (days 1, 4, 43, and 46);
- bleomycin: 30 units per day in 1000 cc saline by continuous infusion, daily for 4 days for two cycles only (total dose 240 units); Begun after vincristine on day 1 every 6 weeks (days 1, 2, 3, 4, 43, 44, 45, and 46);
- mitomycin-C: 10 mg/m^2 on day 2 for two cycles only every 6 weeks (days 2 and 44);
- cisplatin: 50 mg/m^2 on days 2, 23, 44, 65, 86, 107, and 128.

Chemotherapy was initiated within 6 weeks of clinical and/or surgical staging. All patients were to receive an adequate trial (i.e. at least 6 weeks or one full course of chemotherapy followed by radiation therapy of curative intent) before being removed from therapy due to lack of objective response. Treatment courses were repeated every 6 weeks depending on recovery from myelotoxicity. Vincristine was omitted if the patient developed severe neuropathy or constipation which did not clear prior to the next dose. Cisplatin was given only if the serum creatinine was < 1.6 mg % and was continued at 3-week intervals throughout the course of radiation therapy. Mitomycin-C dose levels (10 mg/m^2, 7.5 mg/m^2, 5 mg/m^2) were decreased according to pre-treatment myelotoxicity (one dose level reduction – WBC 1000–2000/μl and/or platelets 50,000–100,000/μl; two dose level reductions – WBC < 1000 and/or platelets < 50,000/μl). No dose escalations were allowed.

Table 4. Patient characteristics.

Patient	Age	Stage	Histology	Nodal metastases	Disease status at start of chemoRx
1	37	I B	Poorly diff. squamous	+ pelvic & periaortic	2 × 2 cm posterior friable mass
2	31	I B	Squamous	+ pelvic & periaortic	Large firm lesion
3	57	II A	Squamous	+ common iliac	Lesion 2 cm in total size
4	32	II B	Squamous		Bulky disease
5	45	I B	Poorly diff. squamous	+ external iliac	No measurable disease
6	34	I B	Well diff. squamous	+ external iliac	No measurable disease
7	25	I B	Moderately well diff. squamous	+ external iliac	Bulky barrel lesion
8	71	IV A	Squamous		Large exophytic tumor involving cervix, fornices, and anterior vaginal wall, extending into lower 1/3 of vagina and also involving bladder
9	56	III B	Squamous		Disease extension into L. parametrial area contiguous with sidewall
10	42	III B	Squamous		Bulky cervical lesion extending into both parametria and lower 1/3 of vagina
11	54	III B	Squamous		Bulky disease with involvement of the upper vagina and lower uterine segment; palp. 2 cm obturator node
12	71	III B	Squamous		Large exophytic cervical lesion extending to lower 1/3 of vagina and L. pelvic sidewall
13	64	III B	Squamous		Bulky disease of cervic with L. parametrial mass

Median age = 46.5 years.
Range = (25,71).

Table 4. (Continued).

Patient	Age	Stage	Histology	Nodal metastases	Disease status at start of chemoRx
14	39	III B	Squamous		Large central pelvic mass, lower uterine segment involvement and uterosacral disease to the R. sidewall; total obstruction of R. kidney on IVP
15	30	III B	Squamous		Large ulcerated, necrotic lesion involving almost entire cervix and extending into upper 1/2 of vagina; disease extends to R. sidewall & almost to L. sidewall
16	48	III B	Poorly diff. squamous		Tumor massively involving L. parametrium and extending to L. pelvic sidewall
17	50	III B	Mod. diff. squamous		Circumferential exophytic mass of the cervix; large pelvic mass involving uterus with extension into parametrium & R. pelvic sidewall
18	60	IV B	Adenosquamous		4 cm L. inguinal mass; large friable exophytic mass involving cervix & obliterating upper 1/2 of vagina; extensive nodular mass in pelvis extending to sidewalls
19	38	III B	Squamous		Extensive parametrial disease on R. sidewall
20	59	IV A	Squamous		Sidewall to sidewall involvement; large anterior vaginal wall involvement to the urethral meatus, bladder involvement

Median age = 46.5 years.
Range = (25,71).

Radiation therapy of curative intent was scheduled to start on day 66 and had to begin no later than day 86 following the first day of chemotherapy or at the first evidence of tumor progression during chemotherapy.

Results

Patient characteristics are shown in Table 4. There were five patients (25%) with FIGO stage I disease, two patients (10%) with stage II disease, ten patients (50%) with stage III disease, and three patients (15%) with stage IV disease. Eighteen of the 20 patients entered into this trial had measurable disease. The median age was 46.5 years (range 25–71 years).

Chemotherapy and radiation were well tolerated hematologically; the median nadir WBC was 3,500/μl (range 2,000–6,200/μl), and the median nadir platelet count was 199,000/μl (range 112,000–355,000/μl) (Table 5). Radiation therapy was discontinued in one patient secondary to GI toxicity. Five

Table 5. Hematologic data through radiation.

Patient	No. of courses (MOB+P/P alone)	Nadir WBC (per $\mu l \times 10^3$)	Nadir platelet (per $\mu l \times 10^3$)
1	2 / 3	3.0	237
2	2 / 2	2.6	171
3	2 / 2	3.5	201
4	2 / 3	3.5	185
5	2 / 2	3.9	112
6	2 / 2	3.4	225
7	1 / 1	3.0	154
8	2 / 2	4.0	355
9	2 / 1	3.4	237
10	2 / 2	4.8	197
11	2 / 4	4.7	182
12	2 / 4	3.8	319
13	2 / 2	3.5	199
14	2 / 3	2.2	335
15	1 / 1	*	*
16	2 / 3	2.8	249
17	2 / 4	2.0	112
18	2 / 3	2.3	201
19	2 / 2	3.9	159
20	2 / 2	6.2	188
Median	2 / 2	3.5	199
Range	(1,2) / (1,4)	(2.0, 6.2)	(112, 355)

* Patient received only 1 course Rx and then had blocked ureters; therefore, started radiation therapy and experienced tumor growth on radiation.

patients experienced late radiation sequelae, and one of these patients died as a result of treatment complications (Table 6).

As shown in Table 7, the overall response rate to chemotherapy prior to radiotherapy in patients with measurable disease was 72% (CR in three patients - 16.6%; PR in ten patients - 55.5%). Three additional patients (16.6%) showed an improved response (i.e. < 50% but > 25% regression in tumor mass). The patients who had no measurable disease from the study start were not evaluated for response. Descriptions of the radiation therapy given to each patient are listed in Table 8. Following radiotherapy, six (86%) of the seven stage I and II patients have no evidence of disease with a

Table 6. Complications from radiation.

Patient	Stage	Complications	Disease status
7	I B	Small bowel obstruction	NED 24 months
12	III B	Bone necrosis	NED 33 months
13	III B	Rectovaginal fistula	Expired without disease
17	III B	Rectovaginal fistula	Expired with disease
18	IV B	Rectovaginal fistula	NED 17 months

Table 7. Response, after MOB plus cisplatin, before radiation therapy.

Patient	Response	Duration
1	Complete	5/17/83–1/15/86
2	Partial	10/4/83–present
3	Complete	6/14/83–present
4	No	
5	No clinical measurable disease	8/11/82
6	No clinical measurable disease	1/3/84
7	Partial	3/2/84–present
8	Improved	
9	Improved	
10	Partial	5/12/82–10/9/82
11	Improved	
12	Complete	9/15/82–present
13	Partial	1/3/83–4/15/85*
14	Partial	3/29/83–2/25/84
15	No	
16	Partial	9/28/83–1/15/85
17	Partial	10/3/83–10/15/84
18	Partial	11/17/84–present
19	Partial	12/4/84–present
20	Partial	12/15/84–12/15/85

* Patient expired with no evidence of disease.

Table 8. Radiation therapy description.

Patient	Radiation given
1	Whole pelvis and periaortic areas – 4500 rads T & Os – 5000 mg h
2	Whole pelvis – 2000 rads T & Os – 7000 mg h
3	Whole pelvis and lower periaortic – 4500 rads T & Os – 3750 mg h
4	Whole pelvis – 4500 rads Syed implant – 4500 rads to point A
5	Whole pelvis – 4500 rads ovoids – 3500 rads surface dose
6	Pelvis – 4500 rads T & Os – 3500 rads to point A
7	External beam – 2160 rads T & Os
8	External beam to whole pelvis – 4500 rads Syed implant – 4500 rads to point A
9	External beam to whole pelvis – 4500 rads Syed implant – 4500 rads to point A
10	External beam to whole pelvis and periaortic 4420 rads to pelvis and lower periaortic 4080 rads to upper periaortic Syed implants × 2 – 4800 rads to point A
11	External beam to whole pelvis – 4500 rads + 900 rads to L pelvis Syed implant – 4500 rads to point A
12	External beam to whole pelvis – 4500 rads Syed implant – 4500 rads to point A
13	External beam to whole pelvis – 4500 rads Syed implant – 4500 rads to point A
14	External beam to whole pelvis – 4500 rads Syed implant – 4500 rads to point A
15	Whole pelvis – 3900 rads
16	Whole pelvis – 4500 rads Syed implant – 4500 rads to point A
17	Whole pelvis and periaortic, 4500 rads Syed implant – 4500 rads to point A Ovoids 2000 rads surface dose External beam boost to periaortic area, 1500 rads
18	Whole pelvis and inguinal areas – 4500 rads Syed implant – 4500 rads to point A
19	External pelvic – 4500 rads Interstitial implant – 2400 rads
20	Whole pelvis – 4500 rads Syed implant – 4500 rads

median response duration of 28+ months (range 24+ - 33+ months) (Table 9). One patient has had both local and distant recurrence (Table 10). Of the 13 patients with stages III and IV disease, three (23%) have no evidence of disease with a median survival duration of 17+ months (range 14+ - 33+ months). Nine (69%) of these patients have had local or distant recurrences, or both.

Table 9. Survival and current disease status.

Patient	Start date chemotherapy	Last date follow-up	Survival status	Current disease status
1	3/15/83	11/85	Alive	RD*
2	9/14/83	12/85	Alive	NED 28 mos
3	4/11/83	12/85	Alive	NED 33 mos
4	9/19/83	7/85	Alive	NED 24 mos
5	8/11/82	1/85	Alive	NED 30 mos
6	5/26/83	10/85	Alive	NED 29 mos
7	1/3/84	12/85	Alive	NED 24 mos
8	9/27/82	2/23/84	Expired	–
9	5/13/82	5/10/83	Expired	–
10	3/12/82	1/11/83	Expired	–
11	10/14/82	6/6/84	Expired	–
12	8/23/82	5/85	Alive	NED 33 mos
13	10/11/82	4/1/85	Expired	–
14	1/25/83	4/6/84	Expired	–
15	8/19/83	Unknown	Expired	–
16	8/18/83	7/85	Alive	RD
17	8/24/83	6/1/85	Expired	
18	8/6/84	12/85	Alive	NED 17 mos
19	8/1/84	9/85	Alive	NED 14 mos
20	9/1/84	12/85	Alive	RD

NED = no evidence of disease.
RD = recurrent disease.
* Patient had NED following radical hysterectomy at 23 months to treat local recurrence, then bony metastases occurred at 35 months.

Table 10. Disease recurrence.

	Stages I and II no. of patients (%)	Stages III and IV no. of patients (%)
Evaluable patients	7	13
Local recurrence only	0	3 (23)
Distant metastases	0	3 (23)
Local and distant recurrence	1 (14)	3 (23)

Discussion of cervix cancer studies

The overall results of these primary chemotherapy studies in patients with advanced cervix cancers reveal that the various drug combinations are associated with a high overall rate of objective response (i.e. 67 to 100% response rates). Unfortunately, in all but one of these studies [17] the clinical complete response rate was less than 30%. As has been the experience with primary chemotherapy in patients with stage III and IV head and neck cancers [8, 9], it is likely that only those cervix cancer patients who experience a complete response to chemotherapy will have significant prolongation of survival. Thus, continued effort must be directed toward the development of more effective chemotherapy regimens in the setting of previously untreated patients. The relatively high complete response rate reported by Smith *et al.* [17], using intermediate dose methotrexate plus continuous infusion 5FU and high dose cisplatin, is encouraging and deserves confirmation. The Southwest Oncology Group has initiated a trial of this regimen in previously untreated patients with advanced disease.

Although the cure of advanced cervix cancer requires both the eradication of local, bulky disease and the sterilization of distant micrometastases, clearly, the former must be achieved before the latter becomes a problem of significance, In our trial of primary therapy with MOB plus cisplatin [23] six of the nine responding patients with stages IIIB and IVA disease experienced tumor recurrence in the pelvis with or without evidence of distant metastases. Primary systemic therapy alone may not be capable of definitively debulking these large, often poorly vascular tumor masses. The combined approach of primary systemic chemotherapy plus intra-arterially administered drugs or regional hyperthermia might overcome the extreme resistance of these bulky tumors to standard chemotherapeutic agents. Certainly, the primary intra-arterial chemotherapy trials of Scarbelli *et al.* [21] and Kavanagh *et al.* [20] deserve careful evaluation and long-term follow-up. The proven *in vivo* synergism between hyperthermia and cisplatin [24], the most active single agent in the treatment of recurrent cervix cancer, recommends trials of these combined modalities in the setting of advanced cervix cancer.

The use of primary systemic chemotherapy for the control of micrometastatic disease holds considerable promise. Because of the usually good vascular supply to these disease foci (and consequent facilitation of drug distribution) and their slower acquisition of drug resistance (because of the low mutation rate in these small tumors), chemotherapeutic response is likely to be enhanced at these metastatic tumor sites in comparison to response of pelvic tumor masses. As an example, the most promising aspect of our pilot study of primary therapy with MOB plus cisplatin has been the high, long-term disease-free survival rate of the patients with early stage, lymph node positive disease. Six of seven patients in this category remain free of disease with a median follow-up duration of 27 months (range 24–33 months). Since the overall survival rate for these patients is expected to be approximately 60% [1, 2] it is possible that the MOB plus cisplatin regimen has effectively controlled micrometastatic disease in these patients. Obviously, only well controlled, randomized clinical trials will ultimately document the efficacy of this or any other primary chemotherapy regimen.

As has been discussed in an earlier chapter by Dr Piver, the use of hydroxyurea or other, newer agents as radiosensitizers offers considerable promise in the treatment of advanced cervix cancers. The use of one of these agents with definitive radiation therapy following primary chemotherapy would provide a two-pronged approach to the control of bulky pelvic disease. Future studies should focus on this type of trial design. Unfortunately, the acute or chronic toxicities associated with these combined treatment modalities could limit their efficacy. In the MOB plus cisplatin trial [23] there was a 30% complication rate following radiation therapy in the stage III and IV patients. As seen in Table 6 three patients developed rectovaginal fistulas and one died with no evidence of residual disease. It is alarming that the previously reported complication rate at our institution in advanced stage patients treated with transperineal interstitial implants was approximately one half that observed in the primary chemotherapy trial. The administration of cisplatin at 3-week intervals during radiation therapy also could have increased the risk of these complications. For example, one patient developed severe radiation induced enteritis after only 2160 rad of pelvic irradiation.

It is unlikely that post-irradiation administration of cytotoxic agents will prove useful in the prolongation of disease-free or overall survival duration for advanced disease patients. The relative inactivity of anticancer agents in the treatment of recurrent (i.e. post-radiation therapy) head and neck and cervix cancers suggests that radiation-induced tumor mutations and small vessel damage may cancel inherent drug sensitivity.

On the basis of this review of clinical trial data we can draw several conclusions concerning the use of primary and/or concurrent chemotherapy in patients with advanced cervix cancers who are to undergo definitive radiation therapy:

1. Only complete responses to chemotherapy are likely to translate into prolongations of disease-free and overall survival durations following definitive radiation therapy. Thus, the benchmark for all primary chemotherapy trials must be the clinical complete response rate, not the overall complete plus partial response rate.
2. Patients who present with advanced disease, but low tumor burdens (e.g. stage I or II disease with positive pelvic or para-aortic lymph nodes) are

more likely to achieve a final complete remission with subsequent radiation therapy.
3. Primary chemotherapy with cisplatin containing regimens may lead to increased radiosensitivity and thus increased normal tissue toxicity.
4. Combinations of primary systemic plus pelvic intra-arterial chemotherapy and/or concurrent radiosensitizers may be associated with higher complete response rates than with any of these treatment modalities used alone. Phase I trials should be initiated to determine patient tolerance to various combinations of systemic and intra-arterial drug treatments.

Acknowledgements

This work was supported in part by grants CA1904 and CA23074 from the National Institutes of Health, Bethesda, Md 20205.

References

1. Piver MS, Chung WS. 1975. Prognostic significance of cervical lesion size and pelvic node metastases in cervical carcinoma. Obstet Gynecol 46:507–510.
2. Langlands AO, Hudson CN. 1985. Management of carcinoma of the cervix. In: Cancer of the Female Reproductive System (CJ Williams, JMA Whitehouse, eds). John Wiley and Sons, Chapter 13, pp 193–206.
3. Hong WK, Popkin J, Strong MS *et al.* 1984. Adjuvant chemotherapy as initial treatment of advanced head and neck cancer: Survival data at three years. In: Adjuvant Therapy of Cancer IV. Grune & Stratton, pp 127–133.
4. Carter SK. 1977. The chemotherapy of head and neck cancer. Sem Oncol 4:413–424.
5. Oster MW. 1981. Chemotherapy before radiotherapy and/or surgery for locally advanced squamous cell carcinomas of the head and neck. Arch Otolargyngol 107:297–299.
6. Hong WK, Bromer R. 1983. Chemotherapy in head and neck cancer. New Engl J Med 308:75–79.
7. Al-Sarraf M, Drelichman A, Jacobs J *et al.* 1981. Adjuvant chemotherapy with cisplatinum, oncovin, and bleomycin followed by surgery and/or radiotherapy in patients with advanced previously untreated head and neck cancer: Final report. In: Adjuvant Therapy of Cancer III (S Salmon, S Jones, eds). Grune & Stratton, pp 145–152.
8. Kish J, Drelichman A, Jacobs J *et al.* 1982. Clinical trial of cisplatinum and 5-FU infusion as initial treatment for advanced squamous cell carcinoma of the head and neck. Cancer Treat Rep 66:471–474.
9. Ensley JF, Kish JA, Jacobs J *et al.* 1984. Incremental improvements in median survival associated with degree of response to adjuvant chemotherapy in patients with advanced squamous cell cancer of the head and neck. In: Adjuvant Therapy of Cancer IV. Grune & Stratton, pp 117–125.
10. Rosen G, Nirenberg A. 1984. Chemotherapy for primary osteogenic sarcoma: Ten year evolution, and current status of preoperative chemotherapy. In: Adjuvant Therapy of Cancer IV. Grune & Stratton, pp 593–610.
11. Rosen G, Marcove RC, Caparros B *et al.* 1979. Primary osteogenic sarcoma. The rationale for preoperative chemotherapy and delayed surgery. Cancer 43:2163–2177.

12. Bonomi P, Blessing JA, Stehman FB *et al.* 1985. Randomized trial of three cisplatin dose schedules in squamous-cell carcinoma of the cervix: A Gynecologic Oncology Group Study. J Clin Onc 3:1079–1085.
13. Alberts DS, Young L, Mason N *et al.* 1985. In vitro evaluation of anticancer drugs against ovarian cancer at concentrations achievable by intraperitoneal administration. Sem Onc 12(3) (Suppl) 4:38–42.
14. Friedlander ML, Atkinson K, Coppleson JVM, Elliot P, Green D, Houghton R, Solomon HJ, Russell P, Tattersall HMN. 1984. The integration of chemotherapy into the management of locally advanced cervical cancer: A pilot study. Gynecol Oncol 19:1–7.
15. Hakes T, Wertheim M, Daghestani A, Nori D, Clark D, Lewis J Jr. 1984. Adjuvant chemotherapy for poor risk stage IB/IIA cervix carcinoma patients: A pilot study with cisplatin/bleomycin. Proc Am Soc Clin Oncol (Abstract) 3:171.
16. Valle JC, Rezende MR, Werneck C, Chu C, Figueiredo E. 1985. Neoadjuvant and adjuvant chemotherapy with adriamycin, bleomycin, and cisplatin (ABC) and modified radical hysterectomy in the cancer of cervix, stage III. Proc Am Soc Clin Oncol (Abstract) 4:125.
17. Smith MR, Peters WA, III, Goodman G, Tesh D. 1986. Advanced cervical carcinoma: New strategies. Am J Ob Gyn (in press).
18. Fine S, Sturgeon JFG, Gospodarowicz MK, Dembo AJ, Bean HA, Bush RS, Beale FA, Pringle JF, Thomas GM, Herman JG, Rawlings G. 1983. Treatment of advanced carcinoma of the cervix with methotrexate, adriamycin and cisplatin. Proc Am Soc Clin Oncol (Abstract) 2:154.
19. Belinson JL, Stewart JA, Richards AL, McClure M. 1985. Bleomycin, vincristine, mitomycin-C, and cisplatin in the management of gynecological squamous cell carcinomas. Gynecol Oncol 20:387–393.
20. Kavanagh J, Wallace S, Delclos L, Rutledge F. 1983. Induction intra-arterial (IA) chemotherapy for advanced squamous cell carcinoma of the cervix. Proc Am Soc Clin Oncol (Abstract) 2:154.
21. Scarabelli C, Tumolo S, Campagnutta E, Franchin G, Perin A, Grigoletto E. 1985. Intra-arterial chemotherapy (IAC) in patients (PTS) with primary untreated (U) or recurrent (R) locally advanced cervical carcinoma. Proc Am Soc Clin Oncol (Abstract) 4:114.
22. Alberts DS, Martimbeau PW, Surwit EA *et al.* 1981. Mitomycin-C, bleomycin, vincristine, cis-platinum in the treatment of advanced, recurrent squamous cell carcinoma of the cervix. Cancer Clin Trials 4:313–316.
23. Weiner SA, Aristizabal S, Alberts DS *et al.* A phase II trial of mitomycin C, vincristine, bleomycin, cisplatinum (MOBP) as neoadjuvant therapy in high risk cervical carcinoma. Obstet Gynecol (submitted).
24. Alberts DS, Peng Y-M, Chen H-SG *et al.* 1980. Therapeutic synergism of hyperthermia-cis-platinum in a mouse tumor model. J Natl Cancer Inst 65:455–461.

12. Human tumor clonogenic assay studies of cervical cancer

CHARLES E. WELANDER and R. LAMAR PARKER, Jr.

Introduction

The interface between laboratory investigation and clinical oncology remains an area of productive discussion between cell biologists and physicians treating malignancies. Researchers in cell biology have developed techniques for cloning human tumor cells, which now permit *in vitro* studies of fresh human tumors as well as established cell lines. These technical advances have become standardized among laboratories, and a human tumor clonogenic assay (HTCA) now is done on primary human tumors in many centers throughout the world [1–3]. Some types of human tumors have been easier to grow *in vitro* than others. Specifically, cancers of the ovary [4], lung [5, 6], breast [7, 8], and melanomas [9, 10] have been successfully grown in many laboratories, studying the effects of colony formation following treatment with various cytotoxic drugs.

Cancers of the cervix, which are the main topic of this book, have not been one of the 'easy' tumors to grow *in vitro*. Hence, there have not been many reports of tumor growth characteristics or of chemotherapy sensitivity patterns of this tumor type. Nonetheless, there has been some success growing cervical cancers in a clonogenic assay, and these data will be reported in this chapter [11].

This report is divided into three sections, considering application of HTCA techniques to cancers of the cervix. In the first section, clonogenic assay principles and methods will be presented, particularly those modifications of standard laboratory procedures that have been helpful in improving the *in vitro* growth rate of cervical cancers. It is necessary to understand both the realities and the limitations of these HTCA techniques in order to properly apply these laboratory data to clinical problems. The second section covers clinical studies of cervical cancers, looking at effects of cell type on growth *in vitro*, patterns of drug sensitivity of cervical cancers, and application of laboratory data to patient treatment. The last section considers the

E.A. Surwit, D.S. Alberts (eds) Cervix Cancer.

applications of HTCA studies of cervical cancers to investigational drug studies, and to future treatment protocol development.

Clonogenic assay principles and methods

Initial in vitro attempts to study cervical cancers

In vitro growth of human tumors has been a matter of great interest since the early part of this century [12, 13]. Until the availability of antibiotics in the 1930s and 1940s, success with long-term human cell cultures was only anecdotal. In 1952, Dr George Gey of Johns Hopkins University presented his work in which he established a cell line from a human cervical carcinoma which had then been grown *in vitro* for more than 1 year through serial subcultures [14]. This first established cell line was designated the HeLa line, and continues to be used today in basic research.

Over the years since the HeLa line was established, efforts have been continued to establish cell lines of cervical cancers *in vitro*. Technical problems, common to all primary tumor tissue cultures, apply equally to cancers of the cervix. Overgrowth of fibroblasts and other connective tissue elements, which adapt to *in vitro* conditions quickly, will commonly replace the epithelial tumor cells, leaving a culture of only stromal cells. Contamination with vaginal flora from biopsies of cervical cancers will often overgrow in tissue culture flasks, preventing establishment of a cell line. For these reasons, only infrequent successes have been realized in the establishment of long-term cell lines of cervical cancers. One review published in 1975 lists only 11 cervical carcinoma cell lines that have been established in long-term culture [15].

Since the 1950s, cell biologists have attempted to use monolayer tissue cultures of human cancers to determine patterns of sensitivity to cytotoxic drugs. Various endpoints have been selected to measure drug effects on tumor cells *in vitro*. Some investigators reported morphological changes in cells following drug exposure [16]. Others simply counted the number of cells attached to a culture flask after drug treatment. They presumed that drug effects on tumor cells would result in cell death and release of the cell from its attachment to the plastic flask [17]. More recent methods have measured the integrity of the cell membrane after drug exposure, looking at dye exclusion or the release of ^{51}Cr [18]. The uptake of radiolabeled nucleic acid precursors by cells before and after drug exposure has also been used as a measure of drug effect on DNA synthesis [19, 20]. None of these *in vitro* methods can discriminate between cell damage which is temporary, from which repair is possible, compared to effects which render cells incapable of dividing. Likewise, these methods cannot differentiate between drug effects on stromal cells compared to epithelial tumor cells in primary tumor cell cultures. Both stromal and tumor cell populations can grow in monolayer cultures, and can show changes in cell membrane integrity, nucleic acid precursor uptake, etc.

Therefore, it has been of particular significance that primary human tumors can be grown in soft agar cultures, using methods of a colony forming assay described by Hamburger and Salmon in 1977 [21]. The soft agar colony forming assay which has been described exhibits several fundamental biologic principles which are essential, if laboratory data are to be applied to clinical situations. (1) Only malignant cells will form tumor cell colonies in soft agar. Benign stromal elements (in most cases) will not form colonies. (2) Tumor cells from the proliferating compartment (i.e. clonogenic cells) will form colonies in agar. Terminally differentiated cells which are incapable of further cell division will not form colonies. Therefore, 'the cloning efficiency' of a particular tumor sample reflects the number of clonogenic cells in the specimen, which often correlates with the degree of differentiation of the tumor. (3) When cytotoxic drugs are tested in clonogenic assays, only drug effects which render cells nondividing will be measured. Sublethal cell damage from which repair is possible, will not usually result in a decrease in colony formation. In summary, only malignant cells from a tumor specimen, and from the proliferating cell compartment in particular, will form colonies in the HTCA. Hence, the presence of connective tissue stromal elements is not a problem. When antiproliferative drug effects on tumor cells are studied, only those effects which prevent future cell division are measured. Sublethal cell damage is not a confusing factor in endpoint evaluation.

HTCA methods for growing primary cervical cancers

Modifications of the original Hamburger and Salmon technique have been adopted by the Gynecologic Oncology Laboratory at Bowman Gray School of Medicine for growth of primary cervical cancers [11]. Primary tumors received in the laboratory are mechanically minced and washed carefully in saline containing penicillin, streptomycin, and amphotericin B. This is followed by incubation at 37 °C in collagenase and DNAse. Clusters of tumor cells are then incubated in a stirring flask containing hypotonic medium, which serves to disaggregate clusters of cells into a single cell suspension [22]. This cell suspension is then layered over a Ficoll-Paque® gradient, which separates out dead cells and cellular debris, concentrating at the gradient interface viable tumor cells with some other stromal elements present. These are then plated in soft agar as per standard published techniques [11].

An additional modification which has been used in these cultures is the addition of a feeder layer of xenogeneic adherent peritoneal cells from BDF_1 mice. This technique has been described previously [23]. Enhancement of tumor cell growth has been observed in the presence of feeder cells, without changing the patterns of drug sensitivity on these cells.

It has been the policy of the Gynecologic Oncology Laboratory at Bowman Gray School of Medicine to accept for processing only those tumor specimens which can be delivered to the laboratory the same day as removed from the patient. Longer time intervals between surgery and processing the tumor in the lab, as occur when overnight shipping of tumor specimens from remote locations is done, decreases the number of viable cells and the probability of adequate growth *in vitro.*

While many of these technical modifications from the original HTCA description may seem to be trivial, there has been substantial improvement in growth rates of human tumor specimens, using this method. Because the majority of cervical cancer specimens can now be grown successfully *in vitro* with enough colonies to perform drug sensitivity studies, clinical application of such data can be considered.

Clinical studies of cervical cancers using HTCA data

Initial growth rate of cervical cancers in vitro

Biopsy specimens from 99 patients having primary cervical carcinomas were processed by the Gynecologic Oncology Laboratory at Bowman Gray School of Medicine. Methods of specimen preparation for the HTCA are as described previously [11]. Successful growth (defined as > 30 colonies formed in a control culture plate) was achieved in 84 out of 99 patients. Of these tumors, 80 were squamous cell carcinomas, seven adenosquamous,

Table 1. Successful growth of human cervical cancers in a clonogenic assay.

Cell types of specimens received	
Squamous cell	80
Adenocarcinoma	8
Adenosquamous	7
Small cell	2
Other	2
Total	99

Number successfully grown 84/99
(> 30 colonies in controls).

and eight adenocarcinomas. Four patients had miscellaneous cell types, including two small cell carcinomas (Table 1).

Clinical trials using chemotherapy to treat cervical cancers have been reported, showing some activity of cisplatin, bleomycin, mitomycin-C, and vincristine [24–27]. Since these drugs are thought by clinical oncologists to be among the best for treating cervical carcinomas, they have been selected for *in vitro* testing in these primary patient tumor specimens. Each drug has been tested as a single agent by the means of continuous exposure, using two separate drug concentrations. A clinically achievable peak plasma level (PPL) has been determined in patients following an IV bolus injection of a maximal tolerated dose of each drug [28]. A lower concentration, one-tenth PPL, is also tested, to determine whether a greater reduction in tissue levels of a drug will also reduce colony formation in the HTCA.

Since many biopsy specimens of cervical cancers are small and yield limited numbers of viable cells, two concentrations of each of the four drugs were not always possible to test. In order of priority, cisplatin was tested first, followed in sequence by bleomycin, vincristine, and lastly mitomycin-C. There were 84 patient specimens tested with cisplatin, 39 to mitomycin-C, 62 to vincristine, and 75 to bleomycin. In each case a dose dependent response was demonstrated, showing greater inhibition of colony formation when higher concentrations of drug were used (Table 2). Patient treatment results have shown that the greatest clinical predictive capability of the HTCA is seen when colony reduction is demonstrated at one-tenth PPL concentration. If this information is used to select patient therapy, the greatest number of accurate predictions are made.

Attempts have been made to see whether the three cell types included in this study respond differently to each of the drugs. However, the number of

Table 2. In vitro drug sensitivity of cervical cancer specimens.

Drug	Concentration (μg/ml)	No. of specimens tested	% of specimens that show some sensitivity
Cisplatin	2.50	84	38.1
	0.25	45	20.0
Vincristine	0.372	62	33.9
	0.0372	41	19.5
Bleomycin	0.52	75	48.0
	0.052	44	38.6
Mitomycin-C	3.0	39	71.2
	0.3	32	43.8

Sensitivity is defined as reduction in colony survival to less than 50% of controls.

patients with adenocarcinomas or with adenosquamous tumor types is too small to separate them from the much larger group of squamous cell carcinomas.

Clinical application of HTCA data to patient treatment

A small group of 18 patients has been treated with single agent chemotherapy, correlating the results of treatment with HTCA data in a retrospective fashion. The majority of the HTCA results predicted resistance, as was seen by clinical non-responses in 12 patients. There were six patients who had HTCA data predicting sensitivity, but only three out of the six actually showed at least a partial clinical response (shrinkage of tumor > 50% for at least one month) (Table 3).

Given the relatively ineffective drugs that are available for clinical treatment of cervical cancers, it is simple to predict resistance, both *in vitro* and *in vivo*. At least 70–80% of the patients will fail to respond to any single agent chemotherapy regimen. When the HTCA predicts sensitivity of tumor cells to a certain drug, then that information can be used as a good prognostic factor to determine the likely outcome of chemotherapy. The patient's medical condition, performance status, and bulk of tumor being treated will also have a major impact on the treatment results. The effect of prior radiation therapy on the vascular supply of a tumor bed will profoundly affect the ability to deliver cytotoxic drugs in adequate concentrations to tumor cells, becoming another major factor affecting treatment responses. It is possible to observe certain patient situations when unfavorable host factors do significantly outweigh favorable HTCA information, resulting in a poor clinical outcome.

Clinical oncologists can rarely change the host factors that are encountered when a new patient presents for treatment. However, there may be benefit for some patients if the oncologist is able to identify active drugs or

Table 3. Correlations between HTCA predictions and clinical responses to chemotherapy.

	Predictions *in vitro / in vivo*			
No. of patients	S/S	S/R	R/S	R/R
18	3	3	0	12

In vitro criteria $\frac{\text{S} = < 30\% \text{ colony survival}}{\text{R} = > 50\% \text{ colony survival}}$.

In vivo criteria – response = > 50% tumor shrinkage for > 1 month.

conversely, to eliminate consideration of inactive drugs from a treatment plan. In this particular series of cervical cancer patients, 37.7% of the patients had a least one drug showing some degree of cytotoxic activity, with 62.3% percent of the patients have none of the four drugs reported as active. An important point to note is that 'activity' in the HTCA is not equivalent to a patient cure. It is only rarely that our present chemotherapy regimens actually induce a long-term remission or 'cure' patients with advanced cervical cancers.

Many clinical treatment trials combine two or more drugs simultaneously in the treatment of patients with cervical cancers, and thereby achieve higher response rates than with single agents. Additive and/or synergistic drug effects may be seen *in vivo*, but are more difficult to predict in the HTCA. Various reports from other investigators have been published concerning the effect on colony reduction of two or more drugs in the HTCA. Some investigators have shown that additive and synergistic effects can be demonstrated, while others have shown that the best single agent in a multi-drug combination shows the same colony reduction *in vitro* as the combination of two or three drugs shows together [29, 30]. Combinations of drugs in the HTCA have been tested recently, using investigational agents for cervical cancer cells [31]. However, in treatment planning for patients with cervical cancers, only standard chemotherapeutic agents have been tested, each time as a single drug.

The HTCA used for testing investigational drugs

Clinical oncologists have had a keen interest in direct application of HTCA data to patient treatment planning. However, technical and logistic difficulties with the assay preclude easy application to all patients who have tumor surgically removed. Often it is many months or even years following primary surgery before chemotherapy is considered for a patient, making it hard to predict in advance which patients could benefit from drug sensitivity testing. Therefore, it is unlikely that a major application of clonogenic assay technology will be in the area of individual patient testing as an aid to treatment planning. Instead, a greater impact of this *in vitro* technology will probably be in basic biologic areas of tumor cell growth, and studying the pharmacokinetics of investigational new drugs. It is possible from clonogenic assay studies to obtain clues for optimal drug scheduling, drug concentrations, combinations of drugs, and sequencing of drugs, using target cells from cervical carcinomas. In order for repetitive *in vitro* studies to be done which can verify observed scheduling parameters, concentration differences, etc., established cell lines are often used in the HTCA, rather than primary tumor specimens. Large numbers of cells are required for most investigational drug studies, which can be obtained only from cell lines of known cloning efficiency, that are available over an extended period of time, in contrast to surgical specimens which usually are available only once.

The Gynecologic Oncology Laboratory at Bowman Gray School of Medicine has used two established cell lines from human cervical carcinomas (ME180 [32] and CASKI [33] for a group of studies testing investigational agents in the HTCA. A particular interest of the laboratory has been *in vitro* studies of human interferons, Recombinant human interferon alpha$_2$ (rIFNα_2) (Schering Corporation) has been tested with these two cervical cancer cell lines, as well as with primary tumor cells from four patients. As an example of a means to apply clonogenic assay technology to a preclinical question, the following data are presented.

A dose response curve for each cell line with rIFNα_2 has been established first, using clonogenic assay techniques. If reduction in colony growth is the measured endpoint, then there must be a clear relationship of drug concentration to colonies counted over the desired concentration range. In Figure 1 graphic representation is used to show this dose response relationship for CASKI and ME180 to rIFNα_2; in Figure 2 the same type of dose response is shown to doxorubicin. Note the differences in sensitivity of each of these cell lines. Knowing that a dose response to rIFNα_2 and doxorubicin can be demonstrated, combinations of interferon and doxorubicin have been studied. The statistical methods used to evaluate combined drug effects in a clonogenic assay have been reported previously [31]. In summary, under the additivity model, the percent colony survival following exposure to one

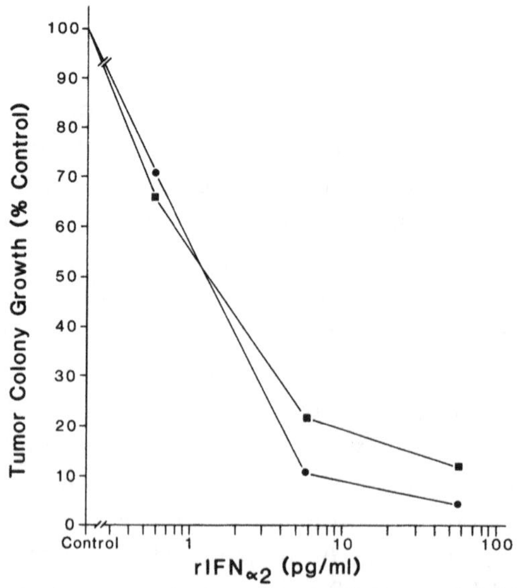

Figure 1. Dose response curve of two cervical cancer cell lines to recombinant interferon α_2, tested in a clonogenic assay. ● = ME180; ■ = CASKI.

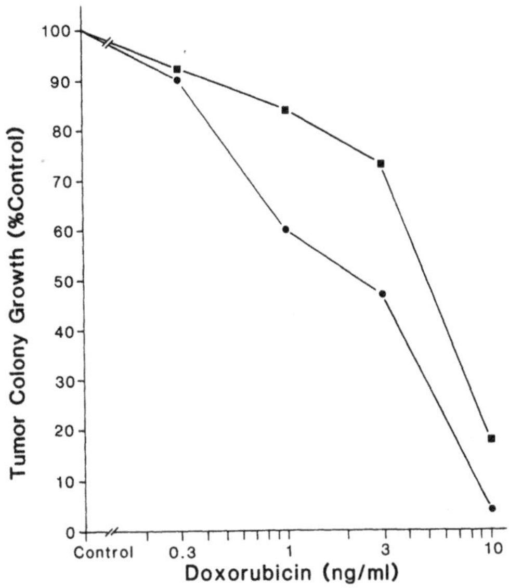

Figure 2. Dose response curve of two cervical cancer cell lines to doxorubicin, tested in a clonogenic assay. ● = ME180; ■ = CASKI.

drug is multiplied by the percent colony survival following exposure to a second drug in order to obtain the 'expected' colony survival. This number is compared to the 'observed' colony survival when both drugs are tested together *in vitro*. When the 'expected' and 'observed' survivals are similar, additive combined effects are being demonstrated. When the observed survival is less than the expected, then synergistic effects are being seen. Subadditive combined effects are described when the observed survival is not equal to the expected survival, but still does show greater colony reduction than either of the drugs alone.

Earlier screening with various malignant cell lines of other tumor types has shown that doxorubicin and cisplatin are two of the most active drugs when tested in combination with rIFNα_2 [31]. Additional earlier studies with various tumor types have shown that exposure of cells to rIFNα_2 prior to or simultaneous with exposure to doxorubicin optimized the observed colony reduction [31]. Therefore, cervical cancer cell lines ME180 and CASKI plus surgical specimens from three patients were tested with sequential rIFNα_2 and doxorubicin (Table 4). The two drugs show synergistic or additive combined effects in most of these cases. It is clear that all cervical cancers are not alike in sensitivity to drugs, suggesting that conclusions based upon the responses seen in a single cell line cannot be used to generalize widely. Further studies have shown that simultaneous combinations of rIFNα_2 and doxorubicin can reduce colony survival in a synergistic fashion, when cell line ME180 or another primary cervical cancer specimen are tested. One further example is of simultaneous combined cisplatin and rIFNα_2, testing one primary cervical cancer. Additive effects were seen in this situation (Table 5).

Tables 4 and 5 are examples of how the clonogenic assay can be used to determine whether certain drugs or combinations of drugs, when tested with cervical cancers, do demonstrate antiproliferative activity or not. If they do show significant *in vitro* antiproliferative effects, then optimal conditions which will maximize these effects can be determined. Using these *in vitro* clues, clinical studies can be designed to treat patients having cervical cancers. This has been done, using combined rIFNα_2 and doxorubicin, written as a phase II clinical trial for cervical cancer patients [34].

Table 4. Sequential treatment of cervical cancer cells with interferon alpha$_2$ followed by doxorubicin.

Cell line or primary tumor	IFN conc. (IU/ml)	Expected colony survival	Observed colony survival	Combined effect
CASKI	100	0.90	0.37	additive
	10,000	0.97	0.06	synergistic
ME180	100	0.80	0.69	additive
	10,000	0.53	0.55	subadditive
Cervical tumor	100	0.84	0.36	synergistic
	10,000	0.89	0.40	synergistic
Cervical tumor	100	0.91	0.70	additive
	10,000	0.81	0.47	additive
Cervical tumor	100	0.32	0.76	antagonistic
	10,000	0.35	0.55	subadditive

Table 5. Combined continuous exposure of cervical cancer cells to interferon alpha$_2$ and doxorubicin.

Cell line or primary tumor	IFN conc. (IU/ml)	Expected colony survival	Observed colony survival	Combined effect
ME180	100	1.31	0.51	synergistic
	10,000	0.77	0.08	synergistic
Cervical tumor	100	1.60	1.29	no effect
	10,000	1.03	0.51	synergistic

Conclusions

Consideration of clonogenic assay studies of cervical cancers cannot go beyond the degree of credibility given to the assay itself. It is necessary to believe that the colony reduction endpoint of the HTCA is related in some way to tumor growth in a patient. Cell biologists have studied human tumor growth in clonogenic assays in sufficient depth to conclude that it is possible to reproducibly grow tumor cell colonies, and to change the colony numbers by varied concentrations of certain cytotoxic drugs. When correlations have been made between *in vitro* predictions and clinical responses, greater than 90% of 'resistant' correlations and 60–70% of 'sensitive' correlations can be predicted [35]. If unfavorable host factors are included in the predictive equation, then even more accurate anticipation of clinical end results is possible. The greatest experience in correlating laboratory and patients results has come from studies of ovarian cancers. Even though ovarian tumors have different growth characteristics and respond to chemotherapy drugs in different ways than do cervical cancers, it seems reasonable to expect that the HTCA can be a useful tool to study human cervical carcinomas as well.

One remaining problem has not been easy to solve. It is known that human cancers consist of heterogeneous populations of cells, which do not all have the same patterns of drug sensitivity. A common empiric clinical means to deal with this heterogeneity of tumors has been to give multiple chemotherapeutic agents simultaneously, attempting to combine non-cross-resistant drugs into a single treatment regimen [36]. It is unexpected that a single drug would be cytotoxic for 100% of the cells in a heterogeneous tumor. Therefore, the HTCA predictions of < 30% colony survival which are empirically defined as 'sensitive' will not be correlated with cures in patients, but only with some degree of clinical response. Studying combinations of drugs in the HTCA has been done with investigational drugs, but is only in the beginning stages of clinical evaluation [31]. If it becomes clear in the future that drug combinations can be tested *in vitro* and that they do correlate well with patient responses, then combinations would need to become a standard laboratory methodology.

As a corollary to the problem of heterogenous tumor cell populations, established cell lines are often not totally representative of primary tumors in patients. While cells from established cultures are always available in greater numbers and for repeated experiments, they are not necessarily a faithful representative of the tumor cell population in the patient of origin. Therefore, *in vitro* studies which draw conclusions from data based only upon cell lines with no primary tumor material, are subject to further verification before they can become credible and be used to build any bridges to clinical problems.

Nonetheless, these data do show that it is possible to grow in the HTCA primary tumor biopsy specimens from 85% of patients with carcinomas of the cervix. The tumor is often accessible to both initial and serial biopsies without significant patient morbidity. While the effectiveness of the presently available armamentarium of cytotoxic agents for treating cervical cancers is discouraging, this fact becomes all the more reason to screen new drugs for treating this disease. It may be that the HTCA can shed light on new agents or on combinations of old drugs which will improve the future for these patients.

References

1. Salmon SE. 1984. Human tumor colony assay and chemosensitivity testing. Cancer Treat Rep 68:117–125.
2. Kern DH, Bertelsen CA, Mann BD, Campbell MA, Morton DL, Cochran AJ. 1983. Clinical application of the clonogenic assay. Ann Clin Lab Sci 13:10–15.
3. Hug V, Thames H, Johnston D, Blumenschein G, Drewinko B, Spitzer G. 1984. The true predictive value of the human tumor stem cell assay: does a workable assay select for treatment responders? J Clin Oncol 2:42–45.
4. Welander CE, Homesley HD, Jobson VW. 1983. In vitro chemotherapy testing of gynecologic tumors: basis for planning therapy? Am J Obstet Gynecol 147:188–195.
5. Kitten CM, Von Hoff DD, Bennett EV Jr, Grover FL. 1982. Growth of lung cancer in a human tumor clonogenic system. J Thorac Cardiovasc Surg 83:363–371.
6. Bertelsen CA, Kern DH, Kaiser LR, Mann BD, Holmes EC, Morton DL. 1983. Biopsy of thoracic neoplasms for assay of chemosensitivity. Arch Surg 118:1074–1076.
7. Sutherland CM, Mather FJ, Carter RD, Cerise EJ, Krementz ET. 1983. Breast cancer as analyzed by the human tumor stem cell assay. Surgery 94:370–375.
8. Sandbach J, Von Hoff DD, Clark G, Cruz AB, O'Brien M. 1982. Direct cloning of human breast cancer in soft agar. Cancer 50:1315–1321.
9. Meyskens FL, Soehnlen BJ, Saxe DF, Casey WJ, Salmon SE. 1981. In vitro clonal assay for human metastatic melanoma cells. Stem Cells 1:61–72.
10. Tveit KM, Fodstad O, Lotsberg J, Vaage S, Phil A. 1982. Colony growth and chemosensitivity in vitro of human melanoma biopsies. Relationship to clinical parameters. Int J Cancer 29:533–538.
11. Parker RL, Welander CE, Homesley HD, Jobson VW, Kawamoto EH. 1984. Use of the human tumor stem cell assay to study chemotherapy sensitivity of cancer of the cervix. Obstet Gynecol 64:412–416.
12. Carrel A, Burrows MT. 1911. Cultivation of tissues in vitro and its technique. J Exp Med 13:387–396.
13. Carrel A, Burrows MT 1911. Cultivation in vitro of malignant tumors. J Exp Med 13:571–575.
14. Gey G. 1952. Tissue culture studies of the proliferative capacity of cervical carcinoma and normal epithelium. Cancer Res 12:264.
15. Fogh J, Trempe G. 1975. New human cell lines. In: Human tumors cells cells in vitro (J Fogh, ed). Plenum Press, New York, pp 115–159.
16. Wright JC, Walker D. 1975. A predictive test for the selection of cancer chemotherapeutic agents for the treatment of human cancer. J Surg Oncol 7:381–392.
17. Berry RJ, Laing AH, Wells J. 1975. Fresh explant culture of human tumors in vitro and the assessment of sensitivity to cytotoxic chemotherapy. Br J Cancer 31:218–227.

18. Roper PR, Drewinko B. 1976. Comparison of in vitro methods to determine drug-induced cell lethality. Cancer Res 36:2181–2188.
19. Shrivastav S, Bonar RA, Stone KR, Paulson DF. 1980. An in vitro assay procedure to test chemotherapeutic drugs on cells from human solid tumors. Cancer Res 40:4438–4442.
20. Volm M. 1981. In vitro short-term test to determine the resistance of human tumors to chemotherapy. Cancer 48:2127–2135.
21. Hamburger AW, Salmon SE. 1977. Primary bioassay of human tumor stem cells. Science 197:461–463.
22. Leibovitz A, Liu R, Hayes C, Salmon SE. 1983. A hypo-osmotic medium to disaggregate tumor cell clumps into viable and clonogenic single cells for the human tumor stem cell clonogenic assay. Int J Cell Cloning 1:478–485.
23. Welander CE, Natale RB, Lewis JR Jr. 1982. In vitro growth stimulation of human ovarian cancer cells by xenogeneic peritoneal macrophages. J Natl Cancer Inst 69:1039–1047.
24. Bonomi P, Blessing JA, stehman FB, DiSaia PJ, Walton L, Major FJ. 1985. Randomized trial of three cisplatin dose schedules in squamous-cell carcinoma of the cervix. A Gynecologic Oncology Group Study. J Clin Oncol 13:1079–1085.
25. Blum RH, Carter SK, Agre K. 1973. A clinical review of bleomycin. A new antineoplastic agent. Cancer 31:903–914.
26. Trope C, Johnsson JE, Simonsen E, Sigurdsson K, Stendahl U, Mattsson W, Gullberg B. 1983. Bleomycin-mitomycin C in advanced carcinoma of the cervix. A third look. Cancer 51:591–593.
27. Alberts DS, Martimbeau PW, Surwit EA, oishi N. 1981. Mitomycin-C, bleomycin, vincristine, and cisplatinum in the treatment of advanced recurrent squamous cell carcinoma of the cervix. Cancer Clin Trials 4:313–316.
28. Alberts DS, Chen HSC. 1980. Tabular summary of pharmacokinetic parameters relevant to in vitro drug assay. In: Cloning of human tumor stem cells (SE Salmon, ed.). Alan R. Liss, Inc., New York, pp 351–359.
29. Alberts DS, Salmon SE, Chen HSG, Moon TE, Young L, Surwit EA. 1981. Pharmacologic studies of anticancer drugs with the human tumor stem cell assay. Cancer Chemother Pharmacol 6:253–264.
30. Sondak VK, Korn EI, Morton DL, Kern DH. 1983. Absence of in vitro synergy for chemotherapeutic combinations tested in the clonogenic assay. Proc Am Assoc Cancer Res 24:316.
31. Welander CE, Morgan TM, Homesley HD, Trotta PP, Spiegel RJ. 1985. Combined recombinant human interferon alpha$_2$ and cytotoxic agents studied in the clonogenic assay. Int J Cancer 35:721–729.
32. Sykes JA, Whitescarver J, Jernstrom P, Nolan JF. 1970. Some properties of a new epithelial cell line of human origin. J Natl Cancer Inst 45:107–122.
33. Pattillo RA, Hussa RO, Story MT, Ruckert ACF, Shalaby MR, Mattingly RF. 1977. Tumor antigen and human chorionic gonadotropin in CaSki cells: a new epidermoid cervical cancer cell line. Science 196:1456–1458.
34. Welander CE, Muss HB, Morgan TM, Trotta PP, Spiegel RJ. 1985. Synergy in vitro and in clinical trials. Inb: Interferon alpha-2: preclinical and clinical evaluation (DL Kisner, JF Smyth, eds). Martinus Nijhoff, Boston, pp 29:39.
35. Von Hoff DD, Clark GM, Stogdill BJ, Sarosdy MF, O'Brien MT, Casper JT, Mattox DE, Page CP, Cruz AB, Sandbach JF. 1983. Prospective clinical trial of a human tumor cloning system. Cancer Res 43:1926–1931.
36. Coldman AJ, Goldie JH. 1982. A mathematical model of drug resistance in neoplasms. In: Drug and hormone resistance in neoplasia, Volume 1 (N Bruchovsky, JH Goldie, eds). CRC Press, Inc., pp 55–78.

Index

www.ingramcontent.com/pod-product-compliance
Lightning Source LLC
Chambersburg PA
CBHW071351220926
51613CB00008B/58
9780898388220